52 Simple Ways
To Health

Carol Phillips

2015

978-0-9906370-0-4 paperback

Second Printing

Published by Health Design LLC
Manchester NH

July 2015

Available as an eBook and paperback
Audiobook available Fall 2015

Cover design: Cindy Estabrook
Page layout: Robin Wrighton
Cover beach photo: © Carol Phillips
Cover portrait photo: www.bstpierrestudio.com

For information, bulk purchase of this book or other products from Health Design, contact: carol@HealthDesignNH.com

www.CoachCarolPhillips.com

Printed in the United States of America

DEDICATION

*This book is dedicated to my parents, John and Pauline,
my children, Cindy and David,
and my entire family.*

Your love and support are priceless to me.

TABLE OF CONTENTS

ACKNOWLEDGEMENTS

My sincere thanks go to all who helped transform this book into an exciting reality, including my loving parents and biggest cheerleaders, John and Pauline Erlman; my supportive, kind, and loving children, Cindy Estabrook and David Phillips; my wonderful family and friends; Chris Biron, who generously contributed to the emergency information section; and my incredibly talented and endlessly supportive book editor, Linda Parker. I would also like to thank everyone who encouraged and inspired me along the way.

PREFACE

Allow me to tell you how *my* story turns into *your* story…

I began my career in health and wellness by teaching countless fitness classes in the 80s and 90s before earning a degree in Exercise Science from Manchester Community College and becoming a Certified Personal Trainer. I loved that work but realized I was working with only one person at a time, and each person was already motivated to make healthy changes, having committed to hiring a personal trainer. I wanted to help thousands, perhaps millions, of people who were struggling to get off that darn couch.

At the time, I was working for the State of New Hampshire. Governor John Lynch issued an Executive Order directing all State agencies to appoint a Wellness Coordinator who would be responsible to promote health and wellness to state government employees and their families. I was privileged to be offered the position at my agency and eagerly began creating seminars and fielding questions on every health topic imaginable.

One common theme I noticed was that sometimes the employees knew the basic answers to their questions, but they were mostly looking to be *motivated* to make the necessary changes needed to reach their goals. Realizing that health coaching was one of my passions and that our culture was in dire need of this service, I returned to college and earned a degree in Health Education from Plymouth State University.

Since then, I have had the opportunity to help thousands of people through my individual and corporate health coaching, speaking, seminars, workshops, and consulting. Besides the benefit of being able to educate and motivate large numbers of people at one time, I enjoy teaching businesses the value of wellness programs and some of the simple changes they can make to inspire their employees to live happier, healthier and more productive lives. The employee benefits, the employer makes more money when employees are more productive, and health care costs are reduced. It's a win-win-win situation!

One of the skills I teach all of my clients – and I believe this skill is KEY – is that making healthy choices does *not* have to be difficult. In fact, often it can be very easy, especially if you divide the changes into small, easy steps.

The basis of my health coaching is the message that I am not a drill sergeant, and I put the responsibility 100% on my clients. Consequently, I am not pushing them to make the changes; instead, we work together to discover what works for them and what doesn't.

Then, when they celebrate a success, the accomplishment is ALL theirs to enjoy. Celebrating their own achievements is essential to people making healthy changes that will last a lifetime. Otherwise, the healthy behaviors will last only until I stop pushing them.

Sure, the drill sergeant mentality sometimes results in faster progress, but the accomplishments realized in working with a drill sergeant will likely be temporary. The drill sergeant goes away, and the client who has failed to develop intrinsic motivation, of course, slips back into old patterns.

Certainly, that person is more disappointed and frustrated than ever, which inevitably leads to further reduced health for the client. I believe we live in a society where, besides the focus being on instant gratification, there is the presence of a strong message that being healthy is very hard, but we "must do it." I agree we must do it; however, presenting it in that manner motivates no one. And isn't failed motivation counter-productive to helping people improve their health by making permanent lifestyle changes?

Taking small steps to improve your health can be very easy, but here is part of the reason why many people struggle – it's also easy to do NOTHING. We live in a society where people sometimes see things in black and white. They automatically think, "If doing nothing is easy, then doing something must be hard." Unfortunately, this is flawed logic when it comes to people making the decision to live a healthy lifestyle. They picture a mountain they can't climb. They picture having to go from not exercising at all and being out of shape to needing to get off the couch and run 5 miles every morning.

Is this you? If so, here's the great news! Living a healthy lifestyle doesn't have to be a huge project. Make one small, healthy choice at a time, get the ball rolling, and the ball will pick up speed on its own. One step building on another reminds me of the joke, *"How do you eat an elephant?"* Answer, *"One bite at a time."* One step at a time is the realistic, doable way you can approach the incredibly important topic of health.

Another analogy I use is to think of healthy and unhealthy choices as being steps on a staircase. Each small, healthy decision you make is one step *up* the staircase; each unhealthy decision is one step *down* the staircase. Any time you need to get "back on track," all you have to do is turn around and take one small step up the stairs. Going down the stairs, so to speak, will certainly bring you closer to having health problems; however, a few steps up the staircase and the view becomes better and better. Remember, if you're facing the bottom of the staircase, all you have to do is turn around and take one small step up to begin moving away from health problems and into a healthier direction.

You CAN start making healthy changes and it doesn't have to be time consuming or difficult. Once you shift your priorities and look for the unlimited opportunities that exist to make better choices, this process can take on a life of its own. Change any negative thinking you currently have regarding all your health choices and turn them into opportunities to improve your quality of life and increase your longevity.

Think about the following: what if those choices were taken away from you right now? What if suddenly you were 100% disabled, and the person taking care of you was making poor decisions regarding your health? Would your thinking and motivation change if you were given the opportunity to be able-bodied again?

Sometimes we take our health for granted until it becomes too late. I don't want that to happen to you. I want this book to be a great tool and an important turning point in your life. Yes, changing your life in long-term and beneficial ways *can* be simple and easy – one small step at a time!

The Seven Dimensions of Wellness

The Seven Dimensions of Wellness is a model used to describe overall wellness. I use it as part of the foundation for my health coaching as a way to teach people that health is more than diet and exercise alone. Every aspect of our lives falls under one or more of the seven dimensions. Becoming aware of this realization can give you a new outlook on the importance of your health and inspire you to prioritize YOU in ways you never imagined.

What is the difference between health and wellness?

Health is the absence of disease and being mentally sound. Wellness is making healthy lifestyle choices and having a sense of contentment in life.

Although some people may believe these two terms are interchangeable, you can see that people may be unhealthy (for example, living with cancer), yet live lives of wellness (being happy and taking care of themselves despite their disease). Conversely, people may have "a clean bill of health," yet they are not well because they make unhealthy lifestyle choices and are highly dissatisfied with their lives.

In this way, people fall into one of four categories:

* Healthy and well.

* Healthy, but not well.

* Well, but not healthy.

* Not healthy and not well.

What category describes you best?

I often refer to Plymouth State University's OSSIPEE Model to describe the Seven Dimensions of Wellness. The following are the seven dimensions and a brief question to describe each:

Occupational Health

Does your chosen profession bring fulfillment and a sense of purpose?

Spiritual Health

Does your belief system regarding your life purpose, religion, soulfulness or higher power add value to your life?

Social Health

Do your relationships with other people help you feel connected and supported?

Intellectual Health

Is your mind used to observe, think critically, be creative and solve problems?

Physical Health

Do you exercise regularly, eat healthy and make good choices regarding self-care to avoid illness and injury?

Emotional Health

Do you handle well your feelings and emotions, such as happiness, sadness, anger, love and frustration, including controlling stress?

Environmental Health

Do you feel connected to the planet, use its resources wisely and avoid toxins?

A quality health coaching program takes all areas of your life into consideration when creating a plan for positive, sustainable change. A comprehensive program designed specifically for you makes it easier to identify how the various components of your health work together and affect each other, negatively and positively. Armed with this knowledge and combined with the capability to identify your strengths and weaknesses, the positive lifestyle and behavior changes you've been seeking become much more easily attainable.

"Life is not complex. We are complex.
Life is simple, and the simple thing is the right thing."

~ Oscar Wilde

INTRODUCTION

52 Simple Ways To Health

Are you tired of feeling you're not making good decisions regarding your health? Is society constantly "in your face" about what you "should" be doing concerning healthy eating, exercise, stress, sleep and other health topics? Do you feel as if getting a grasp on your health is going to take too much time and feels like a mountain you can't begin to climb? I totally understand your position and your desire for your life to be different.

Have you been told you need to lose weight, but you are beyond frustrated with trying to make it happen? Maybe you feel you're doing a good job of taking care of yourself, but you want more information and ideas about how to continue making progress.

*If any of these questions resonate with you,
then this book is for you!*

I've taken what feels like a mountain of information from research, the media and health and wellness experts and broken it down into readable sections designed to educate and motivate you to finally change the way you think about your health. I have tackled this task because after many years as a health coach, I realize that people tend to think about themselves as the "haves" and the "have nots" when it comes to health; people who are taking care of themselves and those who are not.

When people put themselves in the "have not" category, it's very difficult for them on their own to break out of that self-imposed label. And it IS just a label. There are no haves and no have nots. Health is important for everyone, and it doesn't have to be a difficult, boring full-time job.

Health is a right, not a privilege. You deserve to be taking great care of yourself. You deserve the right to have a healthy, energized life and for your new level of well-being to be as easy as possible – even fun!

The information in this book will help you start taking the small steps necessary to get the ball rolling. You can do it – *you deserve it* – and my support is with you every step of the way!

CHAPTER 1

My "52 Challenge" That's About To Become *Your* 52 Challenge

"If you know you're not in a healthy place in life,
turn around and take one step – the other steps will follow."

~ Carol Phillips

I LOVE SHARING THIS "CHALLENGE" with anyone and everyone. I've received wonderful and amazing success stories from my clients who started with this simple technique. Designed especially for people who struggle with change, it's an easy way to start the ball rolling toward better health. Once the ball starts rolling, it picks up speed and people start making changes they previously viewed as unattainable.

Each week, choose one very simple and doable change to make that will improve your health. Select something so easy you can't argue your ability to accomplish it. As examples, add an extra 5 minutes to your walk, go to bed 15 minutes earlier, get up 10 minutes earlier or add an extra scoop of vegetables to your dinner plate.

As you choose a new, easy change to make each week, continue the other changes you've made. Vary the health categories. For example, one week choose something exercise related; the next week choose something nutrition related;

the next week work on stress management. Keep track by making a list you keep in your calendar book, on your phone or on the refrigerator.

One of my clients loves going out to eat and decided the first change he was going to make was to ask for a "to go" container before he ordered his meal at a restaurant. As soon as he received his meal, he divided it in half and put half in the container before he started eating. He quickly discovered that half a meal in a restaurant was enough food for him to feel satisfied.

With that one change, he cut his calories, fat and sodium in half for that meal. The bonus was that he had a meal ready for the next day, and he saved money on his weekly food bill. In addition, he enjoyed not having that 'too stuffed' feeling when leaving a restaurant. One simple change can result in a situation that brings multiple benefits!

Switching from drinking 2% milk to 1% milk may help you lose 5 pounds of unhealthy fat in a year with that one change alone. Taking five minutes of quiet time each day is another easy change that may so significantly improve your outlook that you'll find yourself making more healthy lifestyle decisions.

When you spend time consciously being open to new ideas that are simple and easy, you will begin to notice the numerous opportunities right in front of you. As soon as you become aware of them, write them down so you'll have them for the next week.

Now, what small change can you make starting today?

Can you challenge your family and friends to begin the 52 Challenge with you and turn it into a fun game? You can also incorporate this at your workplace by challenging co-workers to come up with ideas everyone can share. One small healthy decision here and there is what good health habits are all about. You will be surprised at how easy it is to jump on the path leading you to a much better place in your life. After 52 weeks and 52 simple and easy changes, you will definitely notice an improvement in your health!

CHAPTER 2

Remember This Word: Homeostasis

*"Do something today
that your future self will thank you for."*

~ Author unknown

ACCORDING TO MERRIAM-WEBSTER Online dictionary, (www.merriam-webster.com/dictionary/homeostasis) homeostasis is defined as, "a relatively stable state of equilibrium or a tendency toward such a state between the different but interdependent elements or groups of elements of an organism, population, or group." When we're focusing on our body and our health, homeostasis simply means that the body is constantly working to remain healthy or return to health.

Almost everything we do in life either helps our body maintain health (homeostasis) or pulls us in a negative direction, leaving the body to work harder to return to health. Remember, we want to be making choices that make it easy for our bodies to stay healthy, to be in a state of homeostasis.

I once had a person describe homeostasis to me this way: "I like to think of homeostasis as my body literally being in balance and standing straight and strong. When I am tempted to make an unhealthy decision, I think of how it will pull me off balance and weaken me more and more, unless I begin to make healthy decisions again. If I've strayed, it helps me remember that with a few, small healthy decisions, my body will work with me to return to homeostasis."

I sometimes think of homeostasis as a rubber band attached to something; let's say some type of anchor. When I'm making healthy choices, the rubber band is not stretched. However, when I make a choice that's not healthy, the rubber band begins to be stretched away from its anchor. I don't want to continue to make unhealthy choices because eventually the rubber band will break. My body won't be able to handle the stress, and that is when illness and disease will overtake my health and wellness.

The good news is that if I start making healthy choices, the rubber band will be quick to return to the anchor, hence a return to healthiness. The body is a great machine, always working to return to health.

What analogy can you use to remind yourself not to stray too far from homeostasis?

CHAPTER 3

The Best Person To Take Care Of You Is You!

"Dream about what's possible,
then waste no time making the dream come true."

~ *Carol Phillips*

WHEN I WORK WITH A NEW CLIENT, one of the first things I explain is my Toolbox Analogy. This helps people realize they're fully responsible for their own health, with the focus being on the positive. I explain, "My health coaching is going to give you a new toolbox with new tools inside to build your new 'house.' The toolbox contains everything you need to take charge of your health. However, if you don't take out the tools and use them, the house will never be built. I can't build it for you; only you can build it. The good news is that every time you take out one of the tools and use it, the success is all yours, and yours alone to celebrate and enjoy!"

When we celebrate and enjoy our successes, our brains want to repeat the behavior, which is crucial. This great feeling is how we get that ball rolling in the right direction and keep it rolling.

What's really interesting is comparing children's behaviors (from the time they are born until they are, say, two years old) to adults' behaviors. Infants and children are concerned only with themselves and their wellbeing. Their behaviors show they are listening to their gut instincts. They are totally focused on the messages they hear from their inner voices. Infants and children wake when their bodies tell them to wake and sleep when their bodies tell them to sleep. Likewise with sucking, eating, stretching, grabbing, turning over, crawling, standing, sitting, walking and other early childhood development areas. These changes are vital for growth, development and health.

Adults, on the other hand, do not always listen to their inner voices and often make choices that are against what is best for them. When do we, as humans, begin to ignore our gut instincts and talk ourselves out of prioritizing our health? And why? What are the internal and external forces that contribute to this phenomenon that pull us away from health?

The above comparison illustrates the importance of listening to your gut instinct; it is there for a reason. It's that little voice in your head telling you what is best for you and what is not. As humans, we often spend a great deal of time talking ourselves out of listening to our gut instinct. This can get us into trouble very quickly, especially when it comes to decisions that affect our health.

The next time your gut instinct tells you to make a healthy decision, think of it as invaluable advice because that's exactly what it is. Your inner voice, or wisdom, is your best friend, so treat it like one. You'll benefit in ways that will surprise you.

CHAPTER 4

Take 100% Responsibility For Your Health

When you get rid of excuses,
possibilities take their place."

~ Author unknown

START NOTICING EVERY DECISION you make that pulls you away from health and places the blame elsewhere. Taking total responsibility for your health will help you make a huge mental shift, resulting in wonderful changes in your life. For example, instead of saying to yourself, "I ate fast food because the person I was with pulled into the drive-through," pack a lunch or insist on stopping somewhere that will allow you a healthier option. Another example: "I can't find the time to exercise." We don't "find" time; we "make" time. When exercise is a priority in our minds, we will make time for it somehow.

In a University of Minnesota's *Taking Charge of Your Health and Wellbeing* (www.takingcharge.csh.umn. edu/) article titled, "What's My Role?" the subject of taking responsibility for your health is explained using four general points: maintain a healthy lifestyle, become an informed healthcare consumer, partner with your providers and seek help when you need it. These steps point out not only the importance of taking control of your health, but also the importance of learning to advocate for yourself.

Become aware of the specific times you blame other people or life's circumstances for each unhealthy choice you make.

* "If Sue hadn't brought brownies to work…"
* "I'm too tired to go for a walk."
* "My doctor's office is always too busy; I'll make an appointment next week."
* "I have no willpower."

The list is endless. When you decide to take TOTAL responsibility for your health and view excuses as an unacceptable cop-out, you will be more likely to start making better decisions. It doesn't have to happen all at once. Slow and steady wins the race. Once you make the decision not to allow excuses to be your roadblock, you can do amazing things.

What areas in your life are negatively affected by not taking full responsibility for your health? Shifting your mindset to a "no excuses" approach can bring with it the added benefit of feeling in control and empowered, which is how you want to feel about your health and wellness.

Taking full responsibility for your health is an area in which journaling can be of great value. At the end of each day, take a couple of minutes to jot down the times that day when you dismissed the habitual excuses, took responsibility, and made a better decision than you would have previously. End the day with some positive reinforcement that you are slowly on a much better path to health. Knowing that you will write down your accomplishments at the end of the day *for which you will give yourself some kudos* will make the decisions even easier.

CHAPTER 5

Analyze YOURSELF:
Every Choice Begins With A Thought

"It is when we are truly quiet, that we can hear the voice
of who we really are as it echoes our capabilities.
Don't just listen; act."

~ Carol Phillips

THE BETTER YOU KNOW YOURSELF, the better you
can take care of yourself. One of the first things I advise my
health coaching clients to do is begin spending time analyzing
every aspect of their lives. You can easily do this type of self-
analysis, too. Truly learning about yourself includes analyzing
the following:

* Your likes and dislikes.

* Your strengths and weaknesses.

* What motivates you and what turns you off.

* Who supports you when it comes to healthy lifestyle
  choices versus who sabotages your efforts.

* What strategies have worked for you versus what you
  view as roadblocks.

* Anything else that helps you determine what motivates
  you and what doesn't.

After spending several days or weeks completing this exercise, various behaviors that either help or sabotage your efforts toward health will be revealed, creating a great starting point for change. Also, make a list of your strengths and motivators you can draw on when facing new challenges.

Over time, the more you recognize what works for you and what doesn't, the better you can advocate for yourself and slowly make better decisions in all areas of health. Making healthy decisions is not just a matter of willpower; many factors are involved. The better you know yourself, the easier it is to make healthy choices.

The ancient Greek saying "Know thyself" has been analyzed extensively regarding its original, intended meaning. I like to think it ties in perfectly with the importance of knowing yourself well enough to aid you in making habitual healthy decisions.

Do what works for YOU, which can be completely different from what works for others. For example, some people like to count calories, and counting calories helps motivate them to avoid overeating. However, *you* may find counting calories daily to be too tedious. Some people enjoy exercising alone, but *you* may prefer to exercise with other people and socialize at the same time. On the other hand, possibly you enjoy both, depending on your mood. Thinking "outside the box" and not feeling pressured to do what works for other people (while ignoring what is best for you) can help you make great forward strides.

After assigning this task to one of my new clients last year, the feedback she gave me was remarkable. She shared with me that this was the first time she had ever stopped to consider what *she* enjoyed doing and her own strengths and weaknesses. She said, "Up until the time you asked me to begin analyzing myself, I was so focused on the wants and needs of other people in my life, I hadn't realized I was constantly putting myself last. I didn't even know myself nearly as much as I knew the other people in my life and what they wanted and needed. The assignment was life changing for me and helped me see why I haven't been prioritizing my health."

Identify your roadblocks to health. If you find yourself running into the same walls over and over again, stop and analyze why you keep repeating those actions. Take a step back and figure out what is keeping you from making even the simplest choices that lead to good health. Find ways to get around those walls or break them down altogether.

Spend time finding the true root cause of why you're not taking care of yourself in most (if not all) areas of your health. You will then create a new path that will make a huge difference in your life.

CHAPTER 6

Aim For Positive Self-Talk

"The person in the mirror deserves your kindness."

~ Carol Phillips

SELF-TALK REFERS TO THE MESSAGES we give ourselves mentally, our mindset about ourselves. For example, if you look at yourself in the mirror, what are your thoughts about your appearance? Are you often highly critical or do you think something positive? If you're working on a project and you make a mistake, do you immediately chastise yourself or is your mental reaction one of self-forgiveness?

Spend a few days paying attention to all of the messages you give yourself. Are the majority of the messages positive or negative? Supportive or critical? Angry or loving?

Next, begin to look for patterns regarding which situations help you to be kind to yourself versus the situations in which you don't cut yourself some slack. What thoughts are truly justified and which ones involve self-sabotage?

Self-talk plays an important role in our overall happiness and wellness. If we have a good life but have strong habits of negative self-talk, our lives can be hugely impacted, and many of our decisions can be pulled in a negative direction. For example, if you're trying to eat healthier and you practice positive self-talk, you are much more likely to make choices that help you move in a positive direction. Avoid sending yourself negative messages that will make it easier to choose unhealthy foods.

Changing your self-talk can take time and practice. Habits that we have had since we were very young can be hard to break, but many people have been successful in recognizing their negative self-talk and, over time, consciously finding ways to change to positive self-talk. Feeding yourself those good messages will give you a new outlook on life, reduce stress and bring countless benefits.

An August 2012, article published by Mayo Clinic and titled, "Self-talk: What are you telling yourself?" (www.mayo clinic.org/diseases-conditions/diabetes/expert-blog/self-talk/bgp-20056570) offered some effective ways to break the cycle of negative self-talk, including spending time with people who are positive thinkers, avoiding negative people and environments and distracting yourself with a pleasant activity, such as writing in a gratitude journal. The article also pointed out that negative self-talk may be a sign of depression in certain individuals.

Years ago, when I first learned about self-talk, I was going through a difficult time in my life. I decided to start being conscious of my self-talk. I was surprised to discover that my own self-talk was very negative, very self-critical. I was not at all happy with what I was "hearing" and decided to make a plan to change it. My plan was to catch each time I was giving myself a negative message. Whenever I caught myself, I would say to myself, "Stop!" then I changed the message to something positive I felt was true about myself.

At first, changing my inner dialogue was harder than I had anticipated. Sometimes, I kept falling back into the negative messages within a minute of stopping and giving myself a positive message. In that case, I really paused and consciously thought about the seriousness of changing my thinking. Over time, pushing myself to change worked wonderfully. Now I give myself many times more positive messages than negative ones, which has a direct impact on my health in many positive ways.

I know that you, too, can switch that dialogue in your head from negative to positive. Start right now paying attention to the messages you feed yourself. Spend a few days just listening. Look for patterns. Are there situations in which you give yourself more negative messages than at other times? Are there people who trigger you to be more self-critical than you normally would be? Likewise, identify the people in your life who help you be kinder to yourself. After evaluating your self-talk for a few days, or even weeks, come up with a plan to change the negatives into positives.

Positive self-talk is vital to health and wellness because people who consistently give themselves negative messages are more likely to make unhealthy decisions. On the other hand, positive thoughts are much more likely to result in healthy lifestyle decisions. Do you have someone you can take this journey with and turn it into a social activity, supporting each other along the way? Whether you do it with others or by yourself, changing your thinking will have a profoundly positive effect on your life.

CHAPTER 7

Hear Ye, Hear Ye! Good Health Is Not About Being Perfect

"Believe you can and you're halfway there."

~ *Theodore Roosevelt*

WHEN I HEAR PEOPLE DESCRIBE what they feel they "should" be doing regarding making healthy choices, their descriptions often include picture-perfect scenarios that are not realistic. When people expect themselves to be perfect, you can easily see why they become discouraged from ever getting started on a path toward health.

We have also become a society of extremes in which people often do not give themselves credit for the healthy choices they *are* making. They often feel they need to get to the other end of the spectrum before they can even begin to feel good about themselves. With this line of thinking, most people's efforts will be stalled quickly.

Are you a perfectionist? It's easy to assume that if people are perfectionists, they will be great at taking care of their health. Sometimes the opposite is true because there is no such thing as perfection, and the inability to reach a perceived ideal can create a situation in which perfectionists procrastinate.

Although they desperately want things to be perfect, their minds know absolute perfection is rarely a reality. Perfectionism can result in procrastination when people end up doing *nothing* instead of doing *something* for fear of the effort not being perfect.

When it comes to health, something is *always* better than nothing. In the November 2003 issue of the *Monitor on Psychology* through the American Psychological Association, the article titled, "The Many Faces of Perfectionism," finds that "perfectionism correlates with depression, anxiety, eating disorders and other mental health problems." (www.apa.org/monitor/nov03/manyfaces.aspx)

Most people are served well by a mental shift that includes consciously making two very important changes. First, take time to recognize the areas of your life in which you *are* making healthy choices. Giving yourself a pat on the back when you make a healthy decision is *much more* motivating than a slap on the wrist when you don't. Second, start a plan of change that is slow and realistic. Gradual changes combined with a supportive and forgiving attitude are much more likely to become positive, lifetime changes. Often, people ask me, "Are small changes really worth anything?" The answer is a big, "Yes!" Small modifications are much more likely to grow and become permanent, healthy lifestyle behaviors than bigger changes that are typically harder to make.

Studies confirm that even small changes can have a major impact on improving a person's health. According to a *Prevention* article titled, "15 Teeny Tiny Changes to Lose Weight Faster," a study published in the *Annals of Behavioral Medicine* (www.prevention.com/author/alyssa-shaffer) found that participants who made one, small weekly change to their diet or exercise program made significantly better progress than participants who followed more traditional efforts to improve diet and exercise, such as fad diets or unrealistic increases in their exercise regimen.

Moderation and small, consistent changes are key. A very realistic goal in which many people find success is based on the 80/20 rule. Make healthy choices 80% of the time and don't beat yourself up about the other 20%. Even if it takes you a year (or two) to get up to 80%, that approach is better than not getter there at all. Focusing on your health and wellness will always be a continual process; making healthy choices most of the time and not expecting perfection can be your ultimate goal.

CHAPTER 8

Embrace Change

"Change always brings secret gifts.
Happily anticipate them."

~ Carol Phillips

CHANGE IS SOMETHING MANY PEOPLE struggle with and resist. Having a "fight or flight" response to change is a losing battle because life is constantly changing and we have little or no control over many of the changes. People who fear inevitable changes they *cannot* control are likely to put a chokehold on the changes in life they *can* control. In both instances, this can negatively affect our health and our relationships due to the chronic stress and negative mindset involved in this way of thinking.

Resisting change can be based on several factors, including fear of the unknown, past experiences, or assuming the worst will happen. However, change is rarely all positive or all negative. Most life alterations automatically come with both positives and negatives; how we handle these changes can play a significant role in our overall health.

Think of people who are constantly worrying about something "bad" happening or worrying about upcoming changes in life, assuming the results will be harmful, tragic or disappointing. They live with a constant level of paranoia that certainly affects their health and robs their life of much joy. Too often, people picture the worst possible outcomes, when in reality, life outcomes usually have a balance of positive, neutral and negative effects.

When we fear change so much that we push it away or turn away from it, we miss many of the positive results we could have enjoyed. Fearing change is much like playing baseball and being afraid of being hit by the ball. If you are ready to catch the ball headed your way, you are more likely to make a great catch and give yourself (and all those who are rooting for you) a reason to celebrate the moment. If you are afraid of being hit and you look away, you are much more likely to be hurt.

Having a positive attitude about change does not mean we are relinquishing control and letting life run over us when negative things happen (and negative things will happen). Instead, being optimistic means we are ready to accept and enjoy the positives but are also ready to deal with the negatives. Surviving the disappointments is accomplished by dealing with the negatives we *cannot* control in a positive, healthy way and changing the negatives we *can* control into better situations.

People who embrace change tend to be positive thinkers, which can reduce chronic stress significantly. People who welcome change and look forward to it automatically feel more in control. Their positive attitude and objectivity make them much more likely to adapt to or change any negatives that occur. Interestingly, people often resist change because they feel a lack of control in the situation, which is ironic because if they embrace change, they will be better able to control certain aspects of life's constant transformations.

Picture two of your friends riding a wave on surfboards. One friend is having fun, enjoying the beautiful fresh air and sun while balancing through the rough spots. The other friend looks stressed and is worried the entire time about falling and being eaten by sharks. Who do you think is enjoying life more?

Where do you fall on this continuum? How do you handle change or the mere thought of situations changing? What is your self-talk before, during and after life events happen? Riding the waves of change, while enjoying the sun on your face and keeping your balance, will enable you to reduce stress and stay on your feet.

CHAPTER 9

Find Ways To Build Your Self-Confidence

"You are capable of much more than you realize. Surprise yourself."

~ Carol Phillips

HOW ARE SELF-CONFIDENCE (also known as self-esteem) and health related? Most people take care of themselves at the same level as the level of their self-esteem. In other words, when we feel better about ourselves, we take better care of ourselves, and naturally, our health improves. When our self-assurance is low, we are much more likely to make choices that pull us away from health because subconciously we don't feel we deserve to take care of ourselves.

There are numerous ways to build your confidence; however, if you are one of the many people who suffer from low self-esteem, please be patient with yourself. More than likely, you've been dealing with this issue for years, and it will take time and effort to raise your self-confidence.

Is nurturing your confidence worth the work? Absolutely! A healthy level of self-confidence will positively affect every area of your life.

Many of the concepts in this book can help you improve your confidence in yourself, but finding the root cause of your insecurity may be helpful. What can you do to take this important step?

Although knowing the root cause can be helpful in moving forward, you can also move forward without that knowledge. Other ideas include reading self-help books, taking a fun class (such as painting or dance), joining an adult amateur sport group, attending support groups or utilizing counseling services. Exercise, especially cardiovascular exercise, is also a great way to increase self-confidence, for it helps release the "feel good" hormones in our brains.

CHAPTER 10

Let Go Of Past Hurts
For The Good Of You

"Be careful what you think,
because your thoughts run your life."

~ Proverbs 4:23

SAYING, "THE PAST IS THE PAST" is easy, but too often, living by this belief is extremely difficult. Painful situations from our past have a way of poisoning our thoughts, which then affect our behaviors, our outlook on life and eventually our health. These painful memories can keep us from thinking positively, living in a state of contentment and making healthy lifestyle choices.

Which past hurts are poisoning your today? Identify them and make a plan to move past them. Take control of making changes for the better. We can't change the past, but we can stop allowing it to negatively affect our today.

We often use the term "baggage," in referring to our woes and hurts. It is very appropriate in this case. Think of past hurts you are holding on to as heavy, useless bags you are *choosing* to carry around every day. Even on the days you aren't focused on the hurts, if you haven't moved past them, your brain knows they're there, and they impact your health.

Make it a priority to cut the baggage out of your life for good in order to be free of the negativity associated with it.

A difficult part of your past keeps its power every time you hit the "Replay" button in your mind. Taking control and hitting the "Delete" button can free you from a painful past event. Use the "Replay" button for positive, happy memories instead.

Sometimes, getting beyond past hurts in our lives includes forgiveness, yet forgiveness is not always easy. The Mayo Clinic article titled, "Forgiveness: Letting go of grudges and bitterness," (www.mayoclinic.org/healthy-living/adult-health/basics/staying-healthy/hlv-20049421) describes exoneration this way: "Forgiveness doesn't mean that you deny the other person's responsibility for hurting you, and it doesn't minimize or justify the wrong. You can forgive the person without excusing the act. Forgiveness brings a kind of peace that helps you go on with life." In some cases, forgiveness is meant to help *you*, not the person(s) who hurt you.

If moving past hurts is too hard for you to do on your own, solicit help from a professional. One thing that has helped many of my clients is determining whether they have an Employee Assistance Program (EAP) at their workplaces or their spouses' workplaces.

EAPs can be a great resource, for they often provide free, confidential services in a variety of areas, such as counseling, legal and financial services and assistance with locating childcare and elder services, to name a few. These benefits usually cover employees, their spouses and family members. Inquire at your workplace to determine what is available to you and your family. Remember, the weak don't seek help; the strong do. Be strong and take back the peacefulness you deserve.

CHAPTER 11

Stop Procrastinating

*"Someday is not a day of the week.
If you say, 'I'm going to lose weight someday,' you'll be making
that same empty statement a decade from now.
Winners have a timeline."*

~ Dr. Phil McGraw

ARE YOU A PERSON WHO PROCRASTINATES in many areas of your life? Is the problem of procrastination only in the area of your health? Procrastination is a habit that can be hard to change, but it *can* be done. If you picture having to make all the changes to your health at once, you are even more likely to procrastinate. Spend some time recognizing the situations in which you procrastinate and think about how delaying action has a negative effect on different areas of your health.

Try to figure out why you procrastinate and then come up with some small changes you can make to get in the habit of taking action instead of putting things off. For example, if you've been procrastinating about making a medical appointment, take a moment to figure out if there is a reason why you don't want to go to the doctor. If you determine that you're not happy with the doctor you are using, maybe it's time to choose a new doctor. If you haven't been making an appointment because you're nervous about finding out something negative about your health, remember that procrastinating may make the situation worse. Often, when we figure out *why* we are procrastinating, it's easier to take action.

In the Association for Psychological Science's *Observer*, the article titled, "Why Wait? The Science Behind Procrastination," states: "In research settings, people who procrastinate have higher levels of stress and lower well-being. In the real world, undesired delay is often associated with inadequate retirement savings and missed medical visits." (www.psychological science.org/index.php/publications/observer/2013/april-13/why-wait-the-science-behind-procrastination.html)

Procrastination in one area of your life spills over into all others, but the good news is that improving it in any one area also helps you break patterns of procrastination in other areas. For example, no one guarantees that committing to scheduling and keeping doctor visits will help you also become better at saving money for retirement, but you have nothing to lose and everything to gain by trying.

Positive reinforcement is important with any healthy change, and chronic or even occasional procrastination is no exception. After you have been successful in taking action and not pro-crastinating, give yourself positive feedback. Also, take note of the different ways you (and others) have benefitted from taking action instead of procrastinating.

Simple tricks to keep you on track can be helpful. These may include putting things you need to do in your calendar or on your "to do" list. Possibly breaking a task into smaller parts can help you get started. Have friends hold you accountable by having them ask for updates. Another idea is to make a deal with yourself that you won't watch your favorite television show until you have a certain task completed.

Whatever works for you is better than continuing to procrastinate. Your health won't wait indefinitely. Every time you succeed in not procrastinating, give yourself positive feedback and be conscious of all the benefits of taking action. Mentally rewarding yourself with praise and elevating your consciousness regarding procrastination will help you reduce or eliminate future procrastination.

I vividly remember a time when I had set aside a day in my busy schedule to clean my basement, which was well overdue to be tackled. I put on old clothes and sneakers and walked downstairs to attack the beast. Once I was standing in front of years of collected "stuff" and stacks of boxes, I froze. My brain became overwhelmed with the huge task ahead of me and started trying *every which way* to talk me out of having to complete this enormous job.

Since I had already learned to think positively, I told myself that backing out was not an option. I also told myself to take a deep breath and just start with one box; ignore the enormity of the mountain and focus on one step at a time. I opened one box and told myself that doing something was going to be better than doing nothing. Before I knew it, I had succeeded in cleaning the entire basement and I was thrilled that I had pushed past the negative, overwhelmed voice in my head. If I had procrastinated, I surely would have ended the day disappointed with myself and with the task still undone.

Start today. The next time you catch yourself procrastinating, encourage yourself to at least do a small part of what you are avoiding. Then, notice how taking action can reduce your stress and positively affect your health. Begin the journey of forming a new habit of *not* procrastinating.

CHAPTER 12

Decide To Be Happy!

"It isn't what you have or who you are or where you are or what you are doing that makes you happy or unhappy. It is what you think about it."

~ Dale Carnegie

HAPPINESS IS A CHOICE. No matter what you are going through in life, you have total control over how you react to everything. Most situations that upset you can be improved dramatically with the simple decision to change your outlook. Sometimes one of the healthiest choices you can make for yourself is recognizing the areas in life that bring you the most joy and designing more time around those activities. What are the areas of your life that cause you stress or boredom that you can reduce or eliminate?

I had a life-changing event many years ago in which I made an unexpected, mental shift to be happy. Afterward, I realized I had spent my entire life, up until that point, letting circumstances decide my level of happiness in various situations instead of simply allowing myself to be happy, *no matter* the situation.

During a very stressful time in my life, there was a day when I had an appointment with someone. When I arrived, I discovered that the person wasn't there, and I thought he had forgotten our appointment. I jumped to the conclusion that I wasn't important enough for him to remember me, and I became very upset.

On my way home, I suddenly realized I had control over whether I was upset or not. For some reason, I made a mental shift and realized I can decide how happy I want to be in any situation. My life changed forever in that moment. Now I fully understand the statement, "Happiness is a choice." (I later discovered that the missed meeting was a simple miscommunication.)

Sometimes feeling happier is simply a matter of noticing times when you're viewing the glass as half empty instead of half full. Changing your thinking can take time and effort, but if that choice results in you being happier and healthier, the time is *very* well spent. With practice, changing your thinking in this manner will help you find multiple ways to increase your joy and reduce your stress.

A wonderful way to fuel your happiness is to focus on what you are grateful for in your life. Gratitude journals have become popular in recent years and can help you focus on the positive instead of the negative. Many people fall into the trap of saying, "I'll be happy when…" and they name a time in the future. If you make it your mission to seek happiness in every day, your life will be tremendously enriched.

Start right now. What are you happy about in this very moment? Acknowledge it and then have your own little private celebration that this joy exists in your life at this moment.

Are you the type of person who will not use a gratitude journal? Here's an easy alternative: choose a time when you do the same activity every day. For example, when you are getting dressed in the morning or when you're brushing your teeth at night, use that time every day to remember what you are grateful for and how those blessings have enriched your life.

Take your happiness to the highest level possible each day. Your world around you will change in ways you never imagined and your new attitude will be wonderfully contagious!

CHAPTER 13

Make Time To Laugh

*"A good laugh and a long sleep
are the best cures for anything."*

~ *Irish Proverb*

YOU ALREADY KNOW THAT CHILDREN laugh more than adults do, and whether it is twice as often or ten times as often it doesn't really matter. What matters is that adults are failing to take advantage of the beneficial results of laughter.

I wholeheartedly believe that as a society we are missing having more joy in our lives by not being in more situations in which we naturally laugh. Most people's lives are so busy and stress-filled, there isn't much time to relax and be happy, let alone find things to laugh about on a regular basis.

Granted, children don't have many of the responsibilities that adults have, but that just means we need to focus on gratitude more. It's healthy to find more ways to enjoy life and laugh (and smile) more often. Additionally, when we smile and laugh, our bodies have an alkalizing effect on our pH level (see chapter on pH balance), which contributes bountifully to good health.

Laughter doesn't always have to be left to chance. When I want to watch a movie, and life has been unusually stressful, I consciously rent a comedy because I know it's a healthy decision to help balance the stress in my life. It's impossible to be in the midst of a good belly laugh and stress about the problems of the day. Taking a break from all the challenges in life and adding laughter to the mix can be a very healthy thing to do.

What can you do to create more situations in which you know you'll be laughing and having a good time? Are there people in your life who would make it easy for you to achieve this goal? Remember, the best stomachache is one from too much laughing!

CHAPTER 14

"Sit Up Straight"

"Ignore your health and it will go away."

~ Author unknown

WHO WOULD HAVE KNOWN that our mothers were right when they repeatedly reminded us to sit up straight? Turns out, posture is more important than most people realize. The spine and surrounding core muscles are the foundation of our physical being, much like the foundation of a house. If the foundation of a house isn't solid and strong, the house will not remain healthy and strong.

Our bodies are the same as the house. When we sit/stand straight, our core muscles are engaged, our spines are better able to stay healthy and strong, and our minds take on a more in-control state.

Remind yourself many times a day to sit or stand with good posture until it becomes habit. When our posture isn't good, our bodies are continually dealing with a great deal of physical stress, which is transferred to the rest of the body as it tries to make up for what our foundation is lacking. Strong core muscles are important in that they not only support the spine, but also help bones remain strong. Good posture allows the neck and upper back muscles to relax so they don't become overly tight, which is a common problem, especially when we are sitting at our computers for long periods.

Tony Robbins, the famous speaker and motivator, teaches people the importance of sitting up straight and breathing deeply. This practice brings amazing energy not only to the body, but also to the brain and encourages a positive mindset.

Back pain is one of the top reasons people go to the doctor and emergency room. This condition is also one of the top reasons people miss work, which often involves workers' compensation claims and other associated costs. These costs can lead to financial stress on top of dealing with your injury.

What supports a strong, healthy back? Mainly, your abdominal muscles. One of my favorite exercises for the abdominal muscles, because of the "most bang for your buck" benefit, is bicycle crunches. Remember that any exercise that moves multiple joints at the same time is going to help your core muscles become stronger. I often challenge my clients to add bicycle crunches to their daily routine to keep their core strong, *and now I'm challenging you!*

If you don't have any physical issues that would prevent you from doing this exercise, first choose the same time each day and make bicycle crunches part of your daily routine. You can choose a few minutes before you get in the shower or while you're watching television in the evening.

Start by lying on your back on a hard but comfortable surface with your legs straight. Place your fingertips next to your ears (no clasping hands behind your head because this technique puts excessive stress on your neck). Bring one knee toward your chest and try to bring the opposite elbow to your knee. Return to the starting position. Without pausing, bring the other knee toward your chest and try to touch your opposite elbow. Ideally, your legs should be straight and slightly off the floor.

If extending your legs all the way is too difficult or bothers your lower back, keep them bent closer to your chest. Focus on your breathing so you don't hold your breath. Inhale while you are flexing one leg and exhale when you are flexing the other leg.

Do this exercise every day and watch how, over time, you'll be able to do more and more repetitions, and you'll notice your abdominal muscles becoming stronger and stronger.

If you are a person who likes tracking progress, count your reps each day and write them down. Watch them increase over time. Give yourself a break if there's a day you don't feel well or aren't up to doing as many reps as the day before. Life isn't perfect. The important part is jumping back on track as soon as you feel better.

Because muscle balance is important, also choose an exercise to keep your back muscles strong. When exercising, it's important to maintain muscle balance to ensure opposing muscle groups are equally strong. For example, after working your abdominal muscles, work your back muscles. You want to avoid a situation in which one muscle group is stronger than the muscles on the opposing side, which can increase your risk of injury.

To work your back muscles, a good exercise to do after completing your bicycle crunches is to lie on your stomach with your arms bent and your hands near your head. Lift your head, arms and chest off the floor. Hold for 3-5 seconds, if possible. Return to the starting position. Exhale as you are lifting your upper body off the floor and inhale as you return. Repeat until you are fatigued, as this will challenge the muscles and make them become stronger. When working core muscles, muscle balance is especially important because it can affect posture.

An additional benefit to good posture is that it brings more oxygen to the body. When we slouch, we put pressure on the lower portion of the lungs and tend to take shorter, shallow breaths, thereby limiting our oxygen intake. And speaking of breathing, our next topic is…

CHAPTER 15

Breathe Deeply

*"Take care of your body;
it's the only place you have to live."*

- Jim Rohn

WE CAN LIVE A FEW WEEKS without food and a few days without water, but oxygen is at the top of our critical needs list. Every cell in our body needs sufficient oxygen to remain healthy. One of the ways our body receives an adequate supply of oxygen is through exercise.

When we move enough to increase our heart rate, blood flow is increased to every part of our body, sending precious oxygen to every cell. Conversely, when we are inactive on a regular basis, our cells are starved to receive the amount of oxygen necessary to maintain robust health. Over time, cells, desperate for sufficient oxygen, suffer short-term and sometimes long-term repercussions.

However, the inactivity of a sedentary lifestyle is not the only way we deprive our cells of the oxygen they need. Stress leads to shallow breathing, which further reduces the delivery of oxygen to the cells, and muddles our concentration as our brains struggle to function without sufficient oxygen.

Now breathe deeply, and everything changes. Extra oxygen is delivered to the brain, and we are instantly more alert.

When cells are supplied with a healthy amount of oxygen on a regular basis, the risk of illness and disease is reduced significantly. Adequate oxygenation is one of the many reasons why exercise is so crucial to health. For people who don't exercise (yet), even ten minutes of exercise each day to raise the heart rate and bring oxygen to the cells is considerably more beneficial than no exercise at all.

Think of the choice to be sedentary in this way: without enough oxygen, you are literally, slowly suffocating your cells. Not a pleasant thought, right? Moving your body is the best way to allow your cells to receive the oxygen they need to thrive.

CHAPTER 16

Keep A Water Bottle With You

"Water, air and cleanliness
are the chief articles in my pharmacopoeia."

- Napoleon I

IN THE SAME WAY WE NEED OXYGEN, our cells need adequate water to stay healthy; otherwise, we are living in a constant state of dehydration. Compounding this problem is the knowledge that we don't always feel thirsty when we should be drinking water.

Worse yet is the fact that when we first become dehydrated, our body begins to take fluids from our blood and tissues, and we don't even feel thirsty until we are chronically dehydrated. Chronic dehydration is not a healthy situation, yet some people live this way on a daily basis while their bodies struggle to maintain health.

Symptoms of dehydration can include thirst, constant cravings, fatigue, headaches, dark yellow urine, constipation, dry skin, dry mouth, bad breath, low blood pressure, headaches and dizziness. Over time, this constant state of dehydration can have a major, negative impact on our health. Imagine being able to avoid suffering from any of the above health problems caused by dehydration simply by drinking more water each day.

When we are dehydrated, our bodies go into "survival mode" and hold on to water instead of allowing the body to work the way it's supposed to work by using water to speed cellular activity and flush toxins.

Being dehydrated creates a number of problems, including slowing our metabolism and subsequently reducing the number of calories we burn each day. If you are trying to lose weight, being well hydrated is an easy way to speed up metabolism.

Unfortunately, our bodies aren't always good at letting us know we are dehydrated. Instead, we may think we're hungry and eat more instead of taking in more fluids. When you feel hungry, have a glass of water and wait a few minutes to see if the feeling of hunger subsides.

Purchase a water bottle you like and keep it with you. With it close by, you'll be much more likely to drink an adequate amount of water each day. You'll keep sipping if it's within reach. If you don't like drinking plain water, add a small amount of a quality sports drink for flavor and electrolytes.

Keep in mind the latest health concerns regarding chemicals leaking into food and drinks from plastic containers. I purchase non-disposable water containers that are "BPA Free." Using non-disposable containers also helps reduce the amount of garbage sent to recycling centers or landfills. I've learned to drink (and enjoy) my water at room temperature. Two advantages I have found are: (1) I tend to drink more water throughout the day if my water bottle is right next to me, and (2) the bottle doesn't "sweat" from condensation. What is your preference? Do what works for you – just do it.

We all know the recommendation to drink eight glasses of water per day and that the fluids can come from our food sources, as well, such as soups and fruit. Also remember, the more a person weighs, the more water his or her body needs. In addition, increasing water intake helps with weight loss.

Another way to stay hydrated is to order water when you are in a restaurant, even if you're also ordering something else to drink. When you're travelling, make sure your water bottle goes along for the ride. Remember, it's just as important to hydrate in the winter. Drinking herbal tea is a great way to hydrate and increase health. Being properly hydrated helps the body work the way it is designed to work, including flushing out toxins and burning unhealthy fat.

What other ways can you add more fluids each day that work well with your lifestyle and preferences?

CHAPTER 17

Keep An Insulated Lunchbox With You

"Let food be thy medicine and medicine be thy food."

~ Hippocrates

DO THE VENDING MACHINE MONSTERS call your name at 2:00 P.M. every day? Do you frighten people in the office next to you with the rumblings in your stomach? Well, I have a cure for you. One of my best friends is my insulated lunchbox. I always have it on hand to make it easy to keep healthy snacks, meals and drinks available to avoid becoming too hungry and being tempted to raid the sugar and sodium filled vending machine at work. Having it in my vehicle ensures I'll avoid buying an unhealthy meal when travelling, and it can be a lifesaver when I am stuck in traffic.

First, choose a lunchbox that works for you (not too big, not too small, with features you like) because having a lunchbox you like will encourage you to use it regularly. When I decided to buy one, I had fun looking through all the choices in the store and selecting the one I liked best. I knew the more I liked it, the more likely I would be to use it every day.

Also, choose one that comfortably accommodates your water bottles. Another tip is to have extra cold packs in the freezer in case you forget to take them out of your lunchbox in the evening. You can even turn packing lunches and snacks for the next day into a family event by doing it together. Preparing your lunchbox the day before is also a great way to reduce morning rush stress. Take your stocked lunchbox with you every day, not only to work, but also on long errands during the weekend.

Use your lunchbox to introduce yourself to a wide variety of new, healthy food ideas and then have fun with the endless possibilities. Search the internet for great lunchbox ideas. Numerous websites help parents who want to pack healthy lunches and snacks for their children's lunchboxes. Use the ideas that appeal to you.

Smart choices for healthy snacks include fruits, sliced vegetables, nuts, granola bars, applesauce, yogurt, low-fat cheese, a sandwich cut into quarters and trail mix. Several different small containers of healthy snacks have the added benefit of helping you consume a wider variety of vitamins and nutrients to give your body what it needs.

Get excited about your new lunchbox. Allow yourself to flash back to a time when you were in grade school and looking forward to lunch because you knew you had something yummy waiting for you. Sound silly? Good. Life is often too serious.

CHAPTER 18

Diet Has Nothing To Do With Being Hungry

"Those who think they have no time for healthy eating will sooner or later have to find time for illness."

~ Edward Stanley

WHAT DO THE FIRST THREE LETTERS of the word diet spell? Yes, "die," which is probably not the result you are seeking when you're attempting to be healthier!

We can lose weight and become healthier without EVER having to feel miserable in the process. Often, people think the first step to becoming healthy (and, for most, this involves losing excess weight) is depriving themselves of food. Just the thought of being hungry makes me hungry!

The word diet represents what we consume on a daily basis, not going without food, which is the opposite. Shift your focus to buying and eating healthier foods, and you will automatically eat less unhealthy food. Easier said than done, right?

Sometimes making good food choices is hard to do, but start slowly and find items you like. Healthy eating is not about eating foods you don't enjoy, so joyfully and adventurously experiment with new foods until you find what appeals to you.

Do try foods that, as a child, you might have disliked. Sometimes simply preparing the particular food item or recipe differently can change it from something you didn't like to something you now enjoy. The added benefit is the healthier foods will give you more energy to exercise, so you will be burning more calories. A win-win for sure!

If you follow the latest fad diet, you are almost guaranteed to return to your unhealthy eating habits simply because these types of diets are designed to be temporary. Even if you lose weight with the fad, which is likely because that is the goal, you will almost certainly gain the weight back when you go off the diet. Because you have not learned a new healthful and sustainable approach to eating, you will return to your unhealthy habits.

Going from a fad diet to your old routine until your frustration drives you to try the next fad is a process known as yo-yo dieting. Doomed to fail, yo-yo dieting is both unhealthy for your body and devastating to your self-esteem.

People often ask me how they can resist or limit the amount of unhealthy food they eat when those items are within reach. Relying on willpower alone usually doesn't work, and it's too easy to give in to temptation. A much better choice is not buying those items in the first place. What you don't have, you can't eat. Instead, focus on buying extra food that's healthier, including a variety of healthy foods to snack on when those craving monsters attack and threaten your good intentions. Why be so mean to yourself that you stay within easy reach of your enemy?

CHAPTER 19

Choose Foods Wisely:
Add Healthy Foods

"Don't dig your grave with your own knife and fork."

~ English Proverb

A FANTASTIC GOAL IS TO HAVE a healthy relationship with food, especially because we *need* to eat several times every day. Food is essential to sustaining life, and we have no choice but to engage with it several times a day. Instead of thinking of ways to deprive yourself when it comes to eating, focus on adding foods that are more healthful and slowly crowd out the unhealthful ones.

Rather than working to eliminate unhealthy foods all at once from your diet, which will leave you hungry and suffering with cravings, slowly introduce new healthy foods to your daily choices. Over time, your body will automatically want the healthy foods more and more, and the unhealthy foods will be much easier to reduce or eliminate. The added benefit is that, after a while, the healthy foods will taste increasingly better to you and your body will actually begin to crave them. Baby steps are a huge accomplishment in this area!

The internet is a great place to find countless healthy recipes and reputable sites for learning more about which foods are healthy and why. On some websites, you can sign up for free emails so the information will come directly to you on a regular basis. Another option is to "Like" pages on Facebook that post recipes and information about healthful foods.

You may ask, "Won't planning to eat more food make me gain weight, even if it's healthy food?" Yes, it's true that if we begin to consume extra calories and we don't burn them off each day, theoretically, we will gain weight.

However, what is more likely to happen is that the healthy foods will help you feel full longer and will make you feel better and more energetic. Therefore, you will also have an increase in energy for exercising, which will burn more calories.

Remember, all areas of health affect each other. Healthier choices are likely to result in healthier outcomes. So, rejoice! Add healthier foods to your daily meals and snacks and eliminate the thought of having to be hungry in order to be healthy!

CHAPTER 20

Read Food Labels

"Calories alone are not the enemy. Calories are our energy. Calories from unhealthy food and too many of them are the enemy."

~ Carol Phillips

READING FOOD LABELS is an important element of maintaining health. If you're not familiar with the information on a food label and the meaning of each item, go to www.fda.gov and search for information on food labels. As of this writing, the page is titled, "How to Understand and Use the Nutrition Facts Label."

Refuse to let food labeling daunt you, even if at first it seems overwhelming. You don't have to learn everything all at once. If you get into the habit of reading food labels a little at a time, you'll find it's like learning a song on the radio. When a song is new, you don't download the lyrics and spend hours memorizing them. Over time, you automatically learn them through exposure and repetition.

You can take the same approach with food labels. Keep looking at them and learn a little bit here and there, and before you know it, you'll understand much more about food ingredients and how they relate to health than you did before you started reading them. Simply start reading the food labels when you go shopping, and slowly you will learn which foods contain a higher amount of the ingredients you want to avoid and which foods contain healthier ingredients.

It's helpful to know that ingredients are listed in descending order of the amount of each ingredient. For example, if the majority ingredient of the product is sugar, then sugar will be listed first in the ingredients section.

Know what you're putting into your body. As the saying goes, "You are what you eat." Knowing what to avoid is as important as knowing what healthy ingredients to look for in a product.

Notice what the label identifies as a serving size. Often, people will eat more than the amount listed as a single serving. If that is the case, you need to do the math to figure out how much you are consuming in calories, cholesterol, sodium and other ingredients.

For example, if the serving size is listed as ½ cup, but you eat 1½ cups, then you need to triple the amounts listed on the label. If ½ cup of the product has 125 calories, but you are consuming 1½ cups, you are actually consuming 375 calories. Just as importantly, you have tripled the amount of saturated fat, sodium (salt) and the rest of the ingredients.

Reading food labels is easy once you get accustomed to the language and facts typically shown on them. Labels can be a very important part of making healthier food choices. You can even use mealtime with your family as an opportunity to educate each other on the nutrition in your current meal. You could play a guessing game with the numbers. The sooner young children learn to read and understand food labels, the sooner they can use labels as a tool to monitor their own health.

When I present seminars on basic nutrition, one of the questions I always ask is, "Are calories good or bad (healthy or unhealthy)?" They can be either, depending on the situation. Calories give us our energy. View them as positive, not negative. Without calories, we couldn't move a muscle.

Calories are healthy:

1. When we are eating healthy foods (known as nutrient-dense because they contain a high percentage of nutrition with little or no unhealthy ingredients), *and*

2. When we are not taking in, on a regular basis, more calories than our body is using.

Calories are not healthy:

1. When we are choosing unhealthy foods (known as empty calories because they lack nutrition and often include unhealthy ingredients), *and*

2. When we are repeatedly consuming more calories than what we typically use. The excess calories each day will accumulate and that is when we gain weight.

Start reading those labels a little at a time, and before you know it, you'll be on your way to knowing, at a glance, if the product you're holding is a healthy choice for you.

CHAPTER 21

Carbohydrates (Carbs): Your First Energy Source

"Being healthy is a way of life. It's not just about what you feed your body; it's about what you feed your mind and the social environment you keep. Make healthy food choices, exercise your body and brain, and choose your friends wisely."

~ Steve Maraboli

CARBOHYDRATES ARE OUR FIRST energy source and are important for proper brain function. We need healthy carbohydrates to make glucose for our bodies to use immediately or to store for later use. Healthy carbs include fruits, vegetables, milk products, beans, legumes and whole grain products.

Carbs that should be limited or avoided include soda, cakes, cookies and other items commonly known as "junk food." With this information, you can easily see how carbs are healthy in some situations and unhealthy in others.

During the 1990s and 2000s, low-carb diets became very popular, and some people were able to use them to lose excess weight quickly. However, while it's important to reduce or eliminate unhealthy carbs from your daily food intake, a variety of healthy carbs should remain as the majority of your diet in order to supply your body with the vitamins, minerals and nutrients it needs to stay healthy.

After the low-carb diets became widely popular, some people thought that if low-carb diets were good, then no-carb diets would be better. This is not the case, for we need healthy carbs to maintain health. Some common physical side effects of a no-carb diet include headache, nausea, stomach distress, bad breath, diarrhea and mental confusion. People who try low-carb diets can also experience these symptoms if they lower their intake of carbs suddenly and significantly. Their symptoms are the result of the abrupt increase in burning fat and protein for energy that results from the sudden lack of glucose (our body's sugar) from carbohydrates to burn instead.

Do these symptoms sound as if the body is having a healthy reaction to a dietary change?

In most situations, your body will let you know whether something is healthy for you or not. Listen to your body. It is an amazing machine that will usually tell you what you need to know. When focusing on carbs for healthy weight loss and/or a healthy lifestyle in general, I suggest the following:

∗ Significantly reduce or eliminate unhealthy carbs.

∗ Maintain the recommended amount of healthy carbs.

∗ Increase exercise.

∗ Make changes slowly to allow your body to adapt while minimizing side effects.

∗ For more information, contact your healthcare professional.

According to the 2010 Dietary Guidelines for Americans by the U.S. Department of Health and Human Services, adults should derive 45-65% of their total daily calories from healthy carbohydrates. Of these, 70% should be from fruits and vegetables and 30% from whole grains. Numerous variables can change this amount, including a person's weight, age, gender, health conditions and weight goals.

Changes do not have to happen overnight. Give yourself the gift of time when changing direction and choosing a path to health that works for you.

Some changes can be as simple as becoming aware of when certain produce items are fresh, in season and deliciously ripe, which means they will be at their tastiest, inherently helping motivate you to eat healthier. Slowly adding a wide variety of fruits, vegetables and whole grains to your diet will give your body many of the vitamins and nutrients it needs to work at peak performance.

Have you ever wanted to grow your own garden? This is a great way to increase your intake of vegetables and the enhanced flavor is worth the work, and gardening is good exercise, too. Do you have local farmer's markets in your area? Use them. Recipes often taste much better when fresh, in-season produce is used.

CHAPTER 22

Fats: Your Second Energy Source

*"Sometimes the smallest step in the right direction
ends up being the biggest step of your life.
Tip toe if you must, but take the step."*

~ Author unknown

FATS ARE OUR SECOND ENERGY SOURCE. Fats aid
in the absorption of vitamins and in the maintenance of cell
membranes, among other health benefits. Understanding the
difference between healthy fats (unsaturated fats) and unhealthy
fats (saturated fats and trans fats) is an important part of
making informed choices. Reading food labels can be very
helpful in determining which fats are in the foods you consume.

A few examples of healthy fats and foods that contain healthy
fats include olive oil, canola oil, safflower oil, peanut oil,
salmon, tuna, trout, flaxseed oil and nuts. For the most part,
healthier oils are liquid at room temperature and unhealthy
oils are solid at room temperature. Unhealthy fats commonly
show up in chips, cookies, pastries, fried foods and pre-
packaged foods.

Trans fats are the unhealthiest of all fats, which is why the
Food and Drug Administration (FDA) requires them to be
listed separately on food labels. Keep in mind that if a single

serving size of a particular food contains 0.4 or less grams of trans fat, the FDA allows the company to put zero trans fat on the label. For example, if you ate three servings of a food that contains 0.4 grams of trans fat (even though the label says zero trans fat), you are actually consuming 1.2 grams of trans fat. You easily could consume that sneaky, very unhealthy fat without even realizing!

One way to tell if a product has trans fat is to look for the term "partially hydrogenated oil" in the list of ingredients. Limiting, or preferably eliminating, saturated fat and trans fat is a big step in taking care of your health, for these two fats contribute to heart disease, stroke, diabetes and other health problems.

Beware of food products labeled "Reduced fat." Fat has a salty taste to it. Too often, when the fat is reduced in a product, the amount of salt is increased to make up for the difference in the taste.

Unbelievably, the calories from alcohol are basically equivalent to saturated fat. If you're trying to lose weight, reducing or eliminating alcohol can help you reach your goal faster. The importance of what you drink extends beyond alcoholic beverages; your daily intake of fluids can add significantly to your total calorie count. The choices you make regarding what you drink will take you *toward* health or lead you *away* from it.

Outside of the ongoing debate regarding the health benefits of one glass of wine or one beer a day, alcohol does not contain any nutritional value. Too much alcohol contributes to extra calories stored as fat and to a range of other health problems.

Here's a tip regarding ordering alcohol in a restaurant if your goal is to have only one drink: When you first order, ask the server to also bring you a glass of water and ask him or her to refrain from asking you if you'd like another alcoholic drink for the remainder of your visit. Although you may hesitate to take such a deliberate action, think about your goal of living your healthiest life. Any technique that helps you stick to your plan is worth considering!

Focusing on an adequate amount of healthy fats can help ensure you have enough of the fats your body needs to maintain health. According to the 2010 Dietary Guidelines for Americans by the U.S. Department of Health and Human Services, adults should derive 20-35% of their total daily calories from healthy fats.

What are the sources of most of your daily intake of fat? What small changes can you make to reduce or eliminate the unhealthy saturated and trans fats in your diet and include the recommended amount of healthy unsaturated fat? I like to use my snack choices when packing my lunchbox as a way to focus on choosing healthy fats and avoiding unhealthy fats. Knowing that everything I grab out of my lunchbox when I'm hungry is healthy makes eating exciting and guilt-free.

CHAPTER 23

Protein: Your Third Energy Source

"When diet is wrong, medicine is of no use.
When diet is correct, medicine is of no need."

~ *Ayurvedic Proverb*

PROTEIN IS THE BODY'S THIRD ENERGY SOURCE after carbohydrates and fats. Our bodies use protein primarily to build muscle; however, every cell needs protein to stay healthy. Protein also helps us feel full longer; therefore, it's also great as a snack to bridge the time in between meals. Common protein sources include lean meat, poultry, fish, beans, nuts, yogurt, milk, cheese and eggs.

According to the 2010 Dietary Guidelines for Americans by the U.S. Department of Health and Human Services, adults should derive 10-35% of their total daily calories from healthy sources of protein. On average, adult men should consume 56 grams of protein per day, and women should consume 46 grams. A few examples include:

* 1-ounce nuts: 7 grams

* Hard-boiled egg: 6 grams

* 6-ounce low-fat yogurt: 8 grams

* 1 slice of cheese: 5 grams

* 8 ounces of milk: 8 grams

* 2 ounces chicken: 13 grams

There are countless protein supplements on the market; however, most people who eat even a moderately healthy diet consume adequate protein each day. Most importantly, extra calories from protein will not automatically build more muscle.

At the end of the day, extra protein calories not used will be stored as fat. When making healthy choices, focus on protein sources that are non-meat or lean meat in order to avoid adding too much saturated fat and sodium to your diet.

Snacks with protein are a great way to avoid blood sugar spikes and cravings because protein helps us feel full longer. What protein-rich snacks can you put in your lunchbox each morning?

CHAPTER 24

Fiber: Easily Forgotten But Important To Health

*"You don't have to cook fancy or complicated masterpieces
– just good food from fresh ingredients."*

~ Julia Child

FIBER IS A NUTRIENT our bodies need to aid digestion and reduce the risk of a variety of health problems. Although we technically do not "digest" fiber because the body doesn't break the fiber down and absorb it, fiber is a very important part of our diet. The amount of fiber on packaged foods is listed on the label, which can help you calculate whether you're consuming adequate fiber each day.

The 2010 Dietary Guidelines for Americans by the U.S. Department of Health and Human Services recommends 25 grams of fiber per day for women and 38 grams of fiber per day for men. Most Americans consume an average of only 15 grams of fiber daily. In addition, the fiber they do consume often comes from pre-packaged foods in which fiber is added, which is commonly not a healthy choice. (www.health.gov/dietaryguidelines/)

The two main types of fiber are soluble and insoluble. Soluble fiber dissolves in water and thickens to help slow the digestion of food and help you feel full longer. The thickening of soluble fiber helps control blood sugar and cholesterol. Insoluble fiber does not dissolve in water and has more of a laxative effect on the body, which helps prevent constipation.

Foods that contain a healthy amount of fiber include fruits, vegetables, whole grain products, beans and nuts. Whole grain foods, such as pasta, bread and rice contain much more fiber and nutrients than white pasta, bread and rice do, and they're not as highly processed as white pasta, breads and rice are. Because whole grain products are closer to their natural form, they are healthier for you than the more refined versions.

Fiber is an important part of your diet, and consuming an adequate amount can help you control your weight, in addition to helping reduce the risk of health problems, including heart disease and diabetes. Consuming foods with natural fiber is preferable to relying on foods with added fiber or to taking fiber supplements. Eating high fiber foods helps keep your digestive system working at an optimal level.

Challenge yourself to include the recommended amounts of healthy carbohydrates, fat, protein and fiber into your meals each day. Healthy eating doesn't have to be perfect. If you're moving in the right direction, your body will have the "tools" it needs to keep you as healthy as possible.

What healthy choices are you already making that you can feel energized about and replicate more often? Focusing on what is working and making it happen more often is an easy way to get started. Have you incorporated the 52 Challenge? If so, great! If not, nutrition is a topic where there are endless opportunities to make those simple, doable improvements.

CHAPTER 25

Watch Your Salt Intake

"The more you eat, the less flavor;
the less you eat, the more flavor."

~ *Chinese Proverb*

SODIUM (SALT) IS AN ESSENTIAL PART of our diet. Unfortunately, Americans typically consume far more sodium than is necessary for health, and over time, the high levels of sodium can cause numerous health problems, including high blood pressure. High blood pressure increases a person's chance of heart attack and stroke, among other health problems.

Recommended daily amounts of sodium are 1,500-2,300 milligrams per day maximum. According to the 2010 U.S. Dietary Guidelines, "The estimated average intake of sodium for all Americans ages 2 years and older is approximately 3,400 mg per day," which is much more than the body needs. Current estimates indicate that a whopping 70% of the salt in our diet comes from pre-packaged foods, which can be *very high* in sodium content. (www.health.gov/dietaryguidelines/)

When my clients complain about craving foods (often junk food) high in salt, there are a couple of important ways I address this chronic problem. First, I explain how much salt their bodies need versus how much the typical American consumes and the associated health problems.

Second, I explain that over time, their tongues become desensitized to the taste of salt and need more and more to satisfy the craving. Does this type of desensitization apply to you? If so, I recommend you try this helpful tip that will likely make a huge difference in your food choices. Spend a full week dramatically decreasing (not eliminating) your salt intake and make sure you're adequately hydrated. It's only a week; *you can do it.*

After only one week, you'll notice that foods taste better and some of the salty foods you used to eat now taste too salty and are not as appealing. Lowering your salt craving is exactly the result you want to achieve. When foods taste less appealing, we are more likely to avoid those foods and make healthier choices.

If you aren't ready to reduce your salt intake all at once, find ways to reduce the amount of salt you consume in order to work toward getting into a healthy range. Remember, your body needs a certain amount of salt to work properly, including needing it for muscle contraction, which is vital for exercise. However, most people are consuming amounts that easily create numerous health problems. Are you one of them?

When you consume too much salt, your body retains fluid, which increases your blood pressure. Chronic high blood pressure is a potentially deadly condition because of the increased risk of heart attack and stroke. High amounts of salt can also contribute to diabetes and kidney failure. Here are several ways you can reduce your blood pressure:

* Reduce salt intake.
* Reduce stress.

* Maintain a healthy weight.

* Choose healthy foods.

* Increase exercise, especially cardiovascular exercise.

* Reduce caffeine.

* Stop using tobacco products.

* Reduce or eliminate alcohol.

Here's some great news about reducing high blood pressure: people with high blood pressure frequently return their blood pressure numbers to a healthy range with small, positive changes to their health. For example, if a person needs to lose 50 pounds, his or her blood pressure may return to a normal range after losing just 10-15 pounds and making small changes regarding sodium intake. Allow that good news to help you get started in a healthy direction to get your blood pressure out of a dangerous range, which can literally save your life.

When reducing sodium, beware of pre-packaged foods that list "Reduced Sodium" on the front of the package. Numerous products make this claim but too often, they are not healthy products in other ways, or despite the salt reduction, the item still contains an unhealthy amount of sodium. Note that restaurant meals often contain extremely high amounts of sodium. I advise my clients to visit restaurants' websites to look up nutritional information to determine which meals are healthier choices.

When teaching weight management courses, I often ask the participants to break into groups of 3-4 people. I then give each group a printout of the nutritional values of all the foods offered from several fast food restaurants and restaurant chains. Each group receives a different restaurant.

I then instruct them to work as a team to put together a meal that includes a drink, an appetizer, an entrée and a dessert. Here is the twist: they expect me to ask them to put together the healthiest meal possible for that restaurant. However, I actually ask them to do the opposite. I instruct them to focus on saturated fat and sodium and put together the unhealthiest meal possible. I then ask them to come up with three numbers: the total saturated fat, sodium and calories for their entire meal.

When their meal is ready, I remind them of the recommended maximum amounts of daily saturated fat and sodium for the average adult. The numbers are always shocking. Despite the fact that the average adult should not be consuming more than 1,500 - 2,300 milligrams of sodium per day, the total sodium in meals is often as high as 12,000 milligrams. Moreover, the numbers for saturated fat and calories are just as alarming.

You can do this little experiment, too. Think of a meal you commonly order at your favorite restaurant. Use the nutritional values on the restaurant's website to determine if the meal is helping you move toward health or away from health.

Here's another challenge: Track your sodium intake for three to five days. What did you discover? Some people find they are already in a healthy range. However, if your sodium intake is high, what changes can you start making today to avoid long-term health problems? Experiment with a variety of herbs and spices that can introduce you to new flavors. You may not even miss the extra salt!

CHAPTER 26

Watch Your Sugar Intake

"Eating crappy food is not a reward – it's a punishment."

~ Drew Carey

HOW SWEET IT IS! America has a love affair with sugar. We often use it as a major ingredient in our desserts and as a form of celebration. Think about all the sugar at most birthday parties or the fun trip to the ice cream stand after a day at the beach. Holidays are also full of the sweet stuff – Easter, Halloween and Thanksgiving to name a few.

Although many people (including me) wish sugar was 100% healthy, we are learning more each day of the unhealthy consequences of consuming too much sugar. To give some perspective to the high amounts of sugar commonly found in foods, a regular 12-ounce can of soda contains almost 10 teaspoons of sugar, and several brands of 6-ounce (individual) size yogurts contain approximately 6 teaspoons of sugar.

Besides the products we know that contain high amounts of sugar, such as cakes, cookies, candy and ice cream, the following products can also contain an unhealthy amount of sugar, according to WebMD's article "Sugar Shockers:

Foods Surprisingly High in Sugar": bottled pasta sauce, barbeque sauce, ice tea, juice, applesauce, fruit cups, pudding cups, cereal bars, cereals, and vitamin drinks. (www.webmd.com/food-recipes/features/sugar-shockers-foods-surprisingly-high-in-sugar)

Now research is underway evaluating sugar as a problem associated with health problems such as heart disease and dementia. People with Alzheimer's disease often crave sweet foods, which is sometimes blamed on their sense of taste. However, my theory is that the brain already is addicted to the sugar, and as the brain deteriorates because of the disease, the addiction becomes harder to control, for the brain is losing its ability to manage impulses through reasoning.

Sugar substitutes (artificial sweeteners) can be hundreds of times as sweet as natural sugar and draw some people to them because of their lack of calories as compared to natural sugar. The major concern with these products is that they sometimes contain chemicals that are unhealthy to consume and digest.

As a health coach, when a client asks me if switching from products with natural sugar to products with sugar substitutes is a good idea to save calories, I advise that it is not a good decision because sugar substitutes are often not natural food. You are better off to have extra calories from natural means (within limits) and increase exercise than to consume products that research has deemed potentially harmful.

Your intake of sugar is another aspect of health that is important to track, even short term, in order to determine your level of consumption on a daily basis. What high-sugar products can you eliminate from your shopping cart? What healthy, sweet foods, such as fruit, can you consume instead?

Here's a trick. People are creatures of habit. If they eat cookies, they often grab a specific number of cookies each time. What is that number for you?

Or is it a bowl of ice cream? Try this: the next time, take half of what you usually eat and eat more slowly. You'll find you enjoy it more and you just succeeded in cutting your calories and fat in half. Big changes are great, but small changes are equally as important, and they always beat making no change at all.

CHAPTER 27

Avoid Prepackaged Foods; Focus On Foods With One Ingredient

"It's not that I can't eat that.
I'm making the healthier choice not to."

~ Author unknown

SEVERAL YEARS AGO, I heard the advice, "Try to purchase foods with one ingredient." I thought one-ingredient shopping was a great recommendation, and now I pass it on to my clients. Of course, at first they look at me as if I've lost my mind, but then I ask them to think about it.

If you were going to make a healthy chicken stew and wanted to use fresh ingredients, most of the items in your shopping cart would only have one ingredient each: chicken, potatoes, carrots, onions and all the other yummy ingredients you might add. Doesn't that sound like a refreshingly healthy plan?

The good news is that when you make the mental shift to approach shopping this way, shopping for healthier foods is easier. The *better* news is you will then begin to view unhealthy, pre-packaged foods with a long ingredient list as something you should definitely avoid.

A friend of mine shared with me the changes she was making regarding prepackaged foods. She explained, "I would often purchase boxed dinners (the 'just add meat' kind) to make cooking easier when preparing meals after a long day at work. I used to purchase two boxes that would become our family dinner." The dinner, per serving, had very high amounts of unhealthy fat, sodium and preservatives. The unhealthy ingredients were made worse by the fact that they also contained little nutritional value. She knew she needed to get away from this unhealthy practice, but she also knew her family resisted big changes.

She continued, "I decided to start adding healthy sides such as a vegetable or whole grain rice to the dinner and make one box of the prepackaged meal instead of two. To save time during the week, I'd make a large salad on Sundays and use that as a small side dish with dinner. The leftover salad would last a couple of days for preparing quick meals after work on Monday and Tuesday." She also switched from purchasing white, processed dinner rolls to whole grain bread. Slowly, she worked her family away from unhealthy, prepackaged meals.

Aim to make healthier choices, one step at a time, if your diet needs improvement. Placing high expectations on yourself is likely to create too much pressure and lead to you straying from a healthy lifestyle. Become educated on the dangers of pre-packaged foods and read the labels.

Switching from a pre-packaged food with a high amount of saturated fat, sodium, sugar and preservatives to one that is much closer to the daily recommended amounts is a huge step in the right direction. Change does not have to happen overnight, in fact, slow changes are often most likely to become lasting changes.

CHAPTER 28

Overeating And Emotions

"Food is the most abused anxiety drug.
Exercise is the most underutilized anti-depressant."

~ Author unknown

KEEP A JOURNAL FOR THREE DAYS and record if there are any emotions tied to your eating habits. Are you eating out of boredom? Are you eating because you're stressed? Are you eating because you've been taught to eat everything on your plate even after you're full? Many factors can be at play when eating and emotions entwine.

Do you always eat when you watch TV? Are you rewarding yourself for a job well done? Have you been conditioned that after you work hard at something you deserve to eat something unhealthy? Does eating junk food or something unhealthy give you a rush?

Find ways to get to the root of your emotional issues. One painful event from your past may drive you to emotional eating or you may simply be acting out a learned habit that you have repeated many times over the years. Either way, identifying the issue and deciding to solve the problem in order to move in a healthier direction can be a powerful first step in overcoming emotional eating.

Instead of trying simply to stop the behavior without a change of focus, replace the behavior with healthier food or a different activity. Learn to identify the times when you're tempted to "feed your emotions." Have a different activity available to you. For example, instead of grabbing a bag of chips and sitting in front of the television, grab a handful of nuts or an apple and head out for a quick walk. Make a list of things you can do to change the focus when temptation strikes.

Emotional eating can be a serious problem for certain individuals. Support groups and counselors experienced with eating problems are great resources and are widely available. Your healthcare professional can help you find the best fit for you. Reaching out for help is a wonderful way to take care of yourself.

CHAPTER 29

pH Balance: Why Aren't We Hearing More About This?

"The first wealth is health."

~ Ralph Waldo Emerson

IF YOU HAVEN'T HEARD of the importance of pH balance (acidic versus alkaline) in the body, don't miss this area of health that is so vital to understand! Just as pH balance is important for someone who owns a swimming pool in order to have clear pool water, the pH level in our blood needs to be within a target range for optimal health.

According to the WebMD article, "Alkaline Diets," your blood pH should be 7.35-7.45, which is slightly alkaline. A pH of 0 is totally acidic; 14 is completely alkaline; and 7 is considered neutral. All of our lifestyle choices (food, exercise, stress, smoking, alcohol and other aspects of our daily routines) can affect the pH level in our bodies. (www.webmd.com/diet/alkaline-diets)

An incredibly important factor to know regarding pH is that every whole number change on the scale represents 10 times as much change in acidity or alkalinity. For example, if your pH level is 6.35, your body is *ten times* more acidic than the recommended 7.35 pH level. If your pH level is 5.35, your body is *one hundred times* more acidic than the recommended pH level!

You can find a variety of websites that explain the importance of pH balance in the body and what contributes to our blood being acidic versus alkaline. Most foods, drinks and behaviors known to be healthy (green leafy vegetables, green tea, and laughter for example), fall mainly under the alkaline category, and the foods, drinks, and behaviors that are known to be less healthy (processed foods, soda, alcohol and stress, for example), mostly fall under the acidic category. Most people tend to be too acidic.

Focusing on items that digest leaving an alkaline effect can help improve health. As stated, the pH of blood should be slightly alkaline. The typical American diet and lifestyle behaviors, such as smoking, inactivity and stress, have an acidic effect on the body. Some professionals who work in the area of pH balance in the body also believe cancer thrives in an acidic environment and dies in an alkaline environment.

People who suffer from heartburn, which left untreated can lead to esophageal cancer, can be helped by following a more alkaline lifestyle. Heartburn or acid reflux is just one of many health problems caused or worsened by excessive amounts of acid in the body. I believe pH balance is vitally important to improve health and to avoid the negative effects of too much acid in the body.

Do you know your body's pH level? At-home kits are available to test the body's pH level. What small changes can you make in all areas of health to help your pH stay in a healthy range?

CHAPTER 30

Exercise Is Not A Four-Letter Word

"The body was designed to move."

~ Author unknown

THE BODY WAS DESIGNED TO MOVE, and our good health depends on us moving! Generally, our bodies don't care whether we are doing yoga, Zumba, walking, kayaking or jumping rope with our children or grandchildren. We need to move all of our muscles, tendons, ligaments, bones and joints and elevate our heart rates on an hourly/daily basis.

The most common reason people use for not exercising is lack of time. People often say, "I can't find the time to exercise." We don't find time; we *make time*. We make time to do the things we have put at the top of our priority list.

Let's put the importance of exercise into perspective. I often ask people, "If you would receive a million dollars for walking a mile every day for the next year, would you make the time to do it?" Who doesn't say yes to this question?

Your health should be as high a priority as a million dollars is. If you unexpectedly lost your good health, your perception of the importance of being healthy would change *quickly!*

When I was younger, people didn't own cell phones or computers. After school, we had a snack and went outside to play. After dinner and homework, we went outside again to play until the street lights came on, which was the signal to go home.

My generation didn't grow up constantly hearing that we need to exercise; being active was the culture. For many, it began first thing in the morning with our walk to school. One of the most important differences between society then and society now is that we were naturally drawn to whatever physical activity we enjoyed. We didn't think of it as *needing to* exercise, which automatically puts a negative spin on the idea.

As the years passed, more gyms opened, which is great for exercising during cold or rainy weather and for meeting new people while participating in fitness classes. A gym is also a wonderful opportunity for increasing your health education and working with a personal trainer. However, a paid gym membership also contributed to people slowly painting a picture of the gym as the place they "should be going" rather than an experience that was incorporated seamlessly into their lives. Because the gym is "there" and they are "here," they wind up either not going to the gym or dragging themselves there and resenting it.

Technology, without doubt, plays a part in the problem of widespread inactivity. Constantly checking our cell phones and computers has become an addiction that significantly contributes to our obsession with instant gratification. In many aspects of health, balance is important, and there is much imbalance in our culture today.

I think it's important to recognize the unhealthy path we've taken in our view of exercise. This perspective keeps countless people from exercising because we have created such a negative, boring and difficult view of simply moving our bodies regularly.

I grew up taking dance and gymnastics lessons, playing outside and biking. As a child, I loved to move and I still do. I love walking, running (not so much), biking, hiking and horseback riding. Physical activity is a huge part of my physical and mental health. I'm grateful for the ability to participate in activities I enjoy and for the health benefits that exercise brings me.

I would love for our society to get back to simply having fun and then reaping the benefits of exercise as a by-product of that fun. I invite you to join me to begin to climb out of the huge hole we've dug for ourselves and see the light again!

My hope for you is that physical activity becomes an important, fun and wonderfully stress-reducing part of your life. Exercising on a regular basis will give you countless benefits. You deserve to take your health to the highest level possible.

Not sure where to start? Put on a favorite song and just dance.

CHAPTER 31

Choose Exercises That Are Fun For You

"Physical fitness is not only one of the most important keys to a healthy body, it is the basis of dynamic and creative intellectual activity."

~ John F. Kennedy

IF OUR NUMBER ONE PRIORITY when exercising is making sure we enjoy what we're doing, we are much more likely to exercise on a daily basis. Think of things you would take pleasure in doing instead of thinking of exercise as an obligation. Try new activities to keep your brain from becoming bored.

New physical undertakings have additional health benefits; the new movements force the body to work differently regarding muscle strength and balance, which improves our fitness level. A different mode of exercise also forces our brain to work harder, which stimulates new cell growth. New activities often create new social situations.

Many people tell me, "I have kids now; I don't have time to exercise." Exercise is *absolutely crucial* to good health. I advise people to exercise WITH their children. Being physically active is a necessity for all of you, and doing it as a family teaches your children the enormous value of exercise. Find fun things to do with them that you all enjoy. Modeling the importance of exercise and showing them it is fun is one of the best things you can teach your children.

Make a list of things you enjoy doing or activities you've always wanted to do but haven't done yet. Search the internet for ideas, ask your friends or check magazines for suggestions. Consider this, do you like doing things alone or with other people? Maybe try a little of each for a healthy balance.

Choose the activities that will be the most physically active and put them on your calendar. If you try a new activity, and you find you don't enjoy it, move on to a different one and try again.

Challenge yourself to have as much fun as possible while moving yourself physically. There are so many options in life; don't force yourself to participate in an activity you don't enjoy. Find what you love to do. You deserve nothing less. Instead of choosing *whether* you're going to exercise, choose *what type* of physical activity you're going to love!

CHAPTER 32

Cardiovascular Exercise: Get Your Heart Rate Up

"You are one workout away from a good mood."

~ Author unknown

CARDIOVASCULAR (CARDIO OR AEROBIC) EXERCISE occurs when we move continuously, raising the heart rate and keeping it elevated for a period in order to produce good health benefits. Two of the many benefits of cardio exercise include exercising one of the most important muscles in our bodies, the heart, and burning unhealthy fat. Making time for exercise, especially cardiovascular exercise, produces numerous health benefits.

Benefits of cardiovascular exercise (partial list):

* Increases energy
* Aids joint movement
* Reduces blood pressure
* Reduces heart rate
* Reduces stress
* Increases productivity

* Enhances thought process

* Elevates mood

* Increases longevity

* Reduces risk of illness and disease

* Reduces risk of dementia and other age-related diseases

I use the following analogy to illustrate the numerous benefits of cardiovascular exercise: Pretend a new bank opens in your neighborhood and advertises that for every dollar you deposit into a new account, the bank will deposit $50. How fast would you go to the bank to open an account? The rewards of cardio exercise are just this dramatic. The time and energy we contribute to our cardio exercise pays us back with a long list of health benefits, making cardio exercise an excellent investment in your overall health and longevity.

Cardiovascular activity doesn't have to be performed all at one time each day. Doing cardiovascular activities in ten- or fifteen-minute intervals will still produce benefits. Any cardio activity is more beneficial than continuing to be inactive. Obviously, the more you do (within reason), the more you'll benefit. The key is to do activities you enjoy so that exercise becomes a fun habit and not a chore.

What activities can you incorporate into your daily routine to raise your heart rate long enough to maintain or – better still – improve your health?

CHAPTER 33

Strength Training: Keeping You Independent

"If we are creating ourselves all the time, then it is never too late to begin creating the bodies we want instead of the ones we mistakenly assume we are stuck with."

~ Deepak Chopra

STRENGTH TRAINING HAS MANY health benefits. The two I feel most strongly about are:

1. Strength training keeps our muscles strong enough for us to be independent; allowing us to perform our activities of daily living (ADLs), *and*

2. Strength training helps our bones stay strong. When our muscles contract, they pull on the bone. This activity tells the bone to get stronger in order to keep up with the demand on the muscle.

We want to challenge the muscle with weight, so that the muscle and bone do not weaken. Supply and demand is in full force here. When we exercise and demand our body to rise to the challenge, the body responds by supplying stronger muscles and bones.

Muscle soreness is a common effect of performing new exercises. Unless you really overdo it, think of muscle soreness as something positive, not negative. The soreness is the effect of two conditions: lactic acid, a by-product of exercise (which typically lasts for 24-48 hours), and small tears in the muscle fibers, which will heal with the muscle being stronger than before. Instead of being discouraged by muscle soreness after you've increased your exercise, give yourself positive feedback for taking your fitness to a higher level and drink plenty of water to help flush out toxins and heal the muscle fibers.

To keep our bones strong, we need to do exercises that work all of our muscles in order to apply pressure to all of our bones. For example, if we only work our upper body muscles, the bones in our lower body will not stay as strong and healthy, and there will be an imbalance.

Often, I (half) jokingly ask my young clients who do not exercise, "How old would you like to be when you need help on and off the toilet?" Naturally, they are surprised and say, "Never." I remind them that they need to keep their muscles strong if they want to remain independent in the bathroom well into old age. I add, "If you don't exercise, that day will come sooner rather than later and your bones will weaken early, also."

Any activities that challenge your current muscle strength will provide benefits. The key is to challenge the muscle with more weight than it normally supports while avoiding excessive weight that increases the chance of injury. Common weight training exercises include push-ups, squats, lifting free weights and leg raises. Many cardiovascular exercises, such as tennis, swimming, hiking and walking, have strength training components to them, especially when continued long enough to cause muscle fatigue.

If you're just starting out, avoid the trap of being easily discouraged. Everyone starts somewhere. You can even log your efforts and take satisfaction in watching your ability improve over time.

For example, you may start by being able to do only one push-up, but over time, you can slowly increase that number while giving yourself positive feedback for your effort and your improvements, no matter how small. Think about how you'll feel in a year when you're able to do ten or twenty push-ups in a row. More importantly, you'll be reaping the health benefits!

CHAPTER 34

Stretching: Follow-Up Muscle Care

*"Giving up on a goal because of a setback
is like slashing your other three tires because you got a flat."*

~ *Author unknown*

STRETCHING IS IMPORTANT to reduce the risk of injury and maintain a healthy range of motion for all the joints. When we exercise, our muscle fibers shorten and pull on the bone, making our bones move. If we continue to exercise without stretching, our muscles become shorter, and consequently, our bodies do not retain the proper range of motion, and we have a higher risk of injury. Muscles that have become tight and shortened are one of the reasons why some elderly people walk with a limited range of motion. When we stretch after exercising, the muscles return to the proper length for optimal movement.

Whether we should stretch our muscles before or after exercise is a much-debated topic. I believe the best option is to warm up the muscles gradually before exercise with slow, gentle movements and then stretch immediately after exercise when the muscles are warm and have been shortened by exercise. Stretching the muscles should be done gently to prevent injury. Each stretch should be held for at least 6 to

30 seconds, which enables the brain to allow the muscle to relax and stretch properly.

Going for a massage can also help loosen overly tight muscles. Ask your massage therapist to give you feedback on which muscles he or she feels are too tight, so you can spend extra time stretching those muscles in between visits. Stress reduction is also a great benefit of massage therapy.

Do you stretch on a regular basis? Are there areas of your body that are tighter than others that you can stretch more often? Besides stretching after exercise, a good time to stretch is while you're watching television or talking on the phone. Stretching is a very important part of exercise, and you will realize a great return on investment as you age.

CHAPTER 35

Balance: Keeping You On Your Feet

"The secret of getting ahead is getting started."

~ Agatha Christie

EXERCISING YOUR SENSE OF BALANCE is important because it can mean the difference between slipping and catching yourself versus slipping, falling and becoming injured. In an instant, a fall can negatively affect your health for the rest of your life.

Most of our physical mass is in the upper two-thirds of our bodies. This disproportion creates a situation in which we are constantly at risk of falling and becoming injured.

Avoiding falls becomes more and more important as we age. Many falls by seniors result in broken hips. Unfortunately, the fall is usually the beginning of a downward spiral in the senior's health from which they may never recover. In an article titled, "Human Balance And Posture Control During Standing And Walking," (www.cs.cmu.edu/~hgeyer/Teaching/R16-899B/Papers/Winter95Gait%26Posture.pdf) from the University of Waterloo (Canada), the following research illustrates the fall threat to the senior population:

* Deaths due to falls in the demographic of 80 years old and older are almost as high as motor vehicle accident deaths in the 15 to 29 year old demographic.

* Comparing deaths per 100,000 for these two causes, we find the young group (ages 15-29) has 21.5 motor vehicle accident deaths per 100,000, while the elderly group has 185.6 deaths from falls per 100,000.

The University of Waterloo research appropriately concludes, "Society's concern about the 'slaughter on the highways' of our young people should also be focused on the elderly and their exorbitant death rate due to falls."

To reduce the risk of falling, your time is well spent participating in activities that challenge your balance in order to maintain or improve this important skill. Tennis, skiing, skating, ballet, basketball and hiking are just a few of these activities. Using a stability ball is also a great choice. Even something as simple as standing next to a wall or a chair (in case you need to grab it to regain balance) and standing on one foot and then the other can help you work your balance.

Concern about maintaining or enhancing your balance is a great excuse to try a new physical activity. New modes of exercise challenge the brain and balance more than an activity we are used to doing. What new activity will you choose in order to test and enhance your balance?

CHAPTER 36

Ergonomics: Avoiding Acute
And Chronic Injury

"Shortcuts cut life short."

- Author unknown

ACCORDING TO MERRIAM-WEBSTER ONLINE, ergonomics is "an applied science concerned with designing and arranging things people use so that the people and things interact most efficiently and safely." (www.merriam-webster.com/dictionary/ergonomics)

Addressing the health and safety of workers means designing a job to fit a person in such a way as to reduce or eliminate injury caused by stress on the body, either acute or chronic. Common symptoms and injuries include headache, eyestrain, back pain, neck pain and tightness, carpal tunnel syndrome, bursitis, tendinitis and injuries due to falls.

Millions of workers spend dozens of hours each week sitting at desks in front of computers. Some common recommendations that can be easily implemented in order to reduce the stress on the body include:

  * Sitting, with good posture, in a chair that provides good lower back (lumbar) support.

* Chair height adjusted to allow thighs to be parallel to the floor.

* Feet resting flat on the floor.

* When typing, shoulders relaxed, elbows by the side, forearms are parallel to the floor, and wrists in a neutral position.

* Computer screen at a height in which eyes, looking slightly downward, fall on the top third or middle of the screen.

* If correct positioning at desk leaves feet unable to rest flat on the floor, a footrest can be used to support the feet.

Other types of work should be evaluated to create a workplace as ergonomically correct as possible in order to reduce the risk of injury, including repetitive-use injuries. According to the U.S. Department of Labor's Occupational Safety & Health Administration (OSHA), "Implementing an ergonomic process has been shown to be effective in reducing the risk of developing musculoskeletal disorders (MSD) in industries as diverse as construction, food processing, office jobs, healthcare, beverage delivery and warehousing." (www.osha.gov)

Other problematic situations include:

* Poor lighting
* Tripping hazards
* Extreme noise
* Heavy lifting
* Improper posture
* Dangerous tools

* Toxic chemicals

* Air pollution

In addition to your workplace, ergonomics should be addressed at home regarding repetitive work or hobbies that may create stress injuries. What areas of your life can you address to avoid becoming a victim to this type of acute or chronic stress injury? Prevention in this area can save you from the physical, emotional and financial suffering often caused by these types of injuries.

CHAPTER 37

Avoid The Scale, Use A Tape Measure Instead

"Don't be upset by the results you didn't get with the work you didn't do."

- Author unknown

WHEN CLIENTS ASK ME if they should use a scale, I ask them, "Does using a scale motivate you to make healthier choices, or does it discourage you?" If using a scale motivates them, great! If it doesn't, then I suggest they measure their waist with a tape measure instead. The phrase I like to use is, "The waist doesn't lie."

Using a scale sometimes leaves people feeling frustrated for several reasons. If you weigh yourself too often, the scale can seem confusing because your weight fluctuates during the day based on how much you've eaten, whether you've gone to the bathroom, if you're retaining water and other conditions.

The more common problem with using a regular bathroom scale is that you can't see the difference between your muscle weight and your fat weight. Therefore, if you have started to exercise or increased your exercise, the scale may not show a measurable change because your new muscle has weight to it. This is when the tape measure will be your friend. When you lose unhealthy fat and build muscle, your waist size will decrease. You can also use the way your pants fit as a guide.

If you want to use the scale (for example, if you have a significant amount of weight to lose), I suggest using the scale at the same time of day, such as immediately before breakfast but after you have gone to the bathroom, and not use it more often than once a week. Another option is to invest in a scale that calculates your lean muscle mass versus your fat weight.

In general, regarding weight, evaluate the language you use. People often use the term "weight loss" or say, "I need to lose weight." I prefer the term "healthy weight range" for two reasons. First, healthy weight range creates a mind shift from something negative (being overweight) to something positive (moving toward a goal). Second, knowing your healthy weight range numbers, rather than having one specific number you feel you need to reach, creates less pressure and gives you more flexibility.

Many people aim to return to the weight they were in high school. Your weight as a sixteen-year-old may be a very unrealistic goal for you today. As people's bodies change with age, so does their target healthy weight range. Recognizing this change can eliminate the stress created by trying to reach an unattainable goal.

If you choose to measure your waist with a tape measure, be sure to be consistent in how and when you measure. I suggest measuring your waist first thing in the morning after going to the bathroom but before you eat breakfast. Measure your waist from the belly button, around the small of your back and back to your belly button.

Be sure you're standing up straight and measure immediately after exhaling. Do not hold in your stomach. Record the number and keep a log to make your progress easier to track. Do not measure your waist more than once a week or even once a month in order to avoid being discouraged by daily, natural fluctuations in weight.

There are times during the month that you retain more fluids, which can be discouraging if you're hyper-focused on the number on the scale. In addition, if you're beginning to make positive changes to your intake of healthy fluids each day, the fluids may add weight that should not be viewed as gaining unhealthy weight.

Don't spend time stressing over whether or not to use a scale. Go with your gut (no pun intended) and do what's best for you and your health.

CHAPTER 38

Sleep: Quality And Quantity

*"Early to bed and early to rise,
make a man healthy, wealthy, and wise."*

~ Benjamin Franklin

WHILE MOST PEOPLE CITE UNHEALTHY food choices and lack of exercise as common reasons for health problems, they may overlook how important sleep is as a critical component of good health. You gain numerous direct and indirect benefits from a good night's sleep. When we get into a deep sleep (quality) and sleep enough hours each night (quantity), the body can focus on improving health with important healing and restorative processes that occur while we sleep.

People who sleep well at night are positively affected in these areas: exercise, food choices, weight, productivity, stress, memory and mood, as well as other ways. They are also less likely to become ill, be in an accident or have high blood pressure and other diseases, including cardiovascular disease.

In a WebMD article titled, "The Healing Power of Sleep," research shows that health problems including colds and flu, diabetes, heart disease, mental health and even obesity are linked to a chronic lack of sleep. (www.webmd.com/sleep-disorders/features/healing-power-sleep) As we continue to learn more and more about the importance of sleep, I believe quality sleep will reveal itself to be even more important than we currently know.

If you don't sleep well at night, ask yourself these questions:

* Am I eating immediately before going to bed?

* Am I drinking alcohol in the evening?

* Is my room too light?

* Is my room too warm or cold?

* Are there noises interrupting my sleep?

* Are there pets jumping on and off the bed?

* Am I snoring or possibly have a sleep disorder?

* Is there too much stress in my life?

* Am I exercising enough?

One of my friends was having terrible insomnia, so she went to her doctor to ask for a sleeping pill. At the time, she was 26 years old. The doctor told her to start exercising every day and asked her to determine whether she slept better if she exercised in the morning or in the evening.

He told her that if he wrote a prescription for her at her age, she would likely be on four or five prescriptions by the time she was in her forties. She took his advice, and after a couple weeks, she said she was sleeping like a baby. Exercise can be a great benefit to getting quality sleep.

If you have sleep problems and can't solve them on your own, talk to your healthcare professional. Sleep is a critical component of good health. With certain individuals, sleep studies can be very beneficial to determine the root of the problem and determine a care plan.

CHAPTER 39

Rest / Meditation

"Stop. Close your eyes. Breathe."

~ Carol Phillips

EVEN THOUGH REGULAR EXERCISE is important to health, we also need to balance it with rest. Rest is important, mentally and physically. Our body was designed to move but not from morning to night. Take time to recharge your batteries. Although it's easy to think, "I relax by watching TV," the mind continues to be inundated with information when viewing television. It's important to our health to take a break from all the information input and let the brain process all the data it has received.

I used to think it was simply a coincidence when I would take some time out from all the input we deal with in our lives and would then suddenly come up with a great solution to a problem or a new business idea. Now I realize that the ability to problem solve after rest is the result of my brain having the time to process everything going on in my life, come up with answers and be the creative force it is meant to be, without any distractions to interrupt the process.

Whether you call it rest or meditation, decide what works best for you. We live in a very busy, fast-paced society where people sometimes feel that taking this time for themselves is being lazy or unproductive; however, the opposite is true. We need to balance our busy lives with time for our minds and bodies to catch up and do the important work necessary to keep us strong and independent.

Here's my challenge to you:

Take a survey of your family and friends. Ask them how they relax and what they do to help feel re-energized. What calming activities appeal to you that will create more balance in your life?

CHAPTER 40

Kick The Tobacco Habit, Or At Least Cut Down

*"You can, you should,
and if you're brave enough to start, you will."*

~ Stephen King

BABY STEPS OR COLD TURKEY? Only you can answer that question. Either way, quitting smoking (and other tobacco products) or reducing your tobacco use can be one of the best decisions you make in your entire life.

Tobacco contains over 4,000 (yes, 4,000) known chemical compounds with multiple proven cancer-causing agents. As most people are aware, the list of health problems caused by using tobacco products is very long. The financial cost is also staggering. Each year in the United States, we all share the estimated direct and indirect costs of smoking, which is a staggering $289 billion, according to the Centers for Disease Control and Prevention.

Sometimes people feel discouraged when they've tried to quit multiple times. However, studies show the more you try to quit, the higher your chances are of successfully quitting. The way I help clients quit smoking uses a method I've developed over the last several years, and it's proven quite successful.

It involves tobacco users taking time to analyze every aspect of their tobacco use, including when they use, why they use, how they use, where they use, with whom they use and any other factor they link to smoking or other tobacco usage.

I teach them there are numerous factors involved that contribute to the addiction. For example, the physical addiction, the mental addiction, the emotional addiction, the tactile addiction (having something in your hand often), the oral addiction (the cigarette, pipe, or chew in the mouth) and other ways in which people slowly become addicted to seeing the product as their friend. Through this process, they learn it's not just a matter of willpower.

Once the person spends time learning all the elements of their addiction, I help them "build their personal army" to prepare an attack on the addiction. I have clients decide ahead of time how they are going to deal with the different scenarios involved in their smoking because there are multiple ways to remove themselves from the temptations or overcome that particular scenario. As in most areas of life, the better prepared we are, the more likely we are to succeed.

Other important things to remember when you're quitting:

* Drink extra water, for the body needs extra fluids when it's working hard to heal itself.

* Exercise every day; raising your heart rate can give you the same "rush" as having a cigarette.

* You may cough more often and have more mucous as the body heals. Don't be discouraged by the coughing, as it will get better.

* Begin to identify yourself as a non-smoker instead of telling people that you're "trying" to quit. Reframing your definition of yourself increases your chance of success.

* Avoid alcohol and being around other smokers during this time.

* Remove the toxins from your clothes, furniture, vehicle and so forth, so they won't be present to trigger a craving.

* Brush your teeth more often; it helps remove toxins and helps to satisfy the tactile and oral addictions.

* Spend time with the positive, supportive people in your life and avoid people who will tempt you to return to the addiction.

* Constantly give yourself positive feedback!

While we're on the topic of addictions, are there other unhealthy behaviors such as drinking alcohol in excess, doing street drugs or other addiction-based behaviors that are pulling you away from being healthy? My hope is that the information in this book helps you tap into your strengths and gives you tools you can use to help yourself gradually move to a better place in your life. Most communities have great resources available to guide you in a positive direction. You *do* deserve a better life!

CHAPTER 41

Wash Your Hands Often

"When 'i' is replaced by 'we,'
even 'illness' becomes 'wellness.'"

~ *Author unknown*

PROPER, FREQUENT HAND WASHING can prevent the spread of illness and disease and make a huge difference in your health. The Centers for Disease Control and Prevention's website at www.cdc.gov contains great information on the importance of hand washing for the prevention of illness and disease.

An article found on WebMD, titled, "Prevent Colds with Hand Washing," states: "Amazingly, about 80% of infectious diseases are transmitted by touch. The CDC estimates that up to 49,000 people die from the flu or flu-like illness each year, and another 5,000 people die from food-borne illness each year. And the best protection from this type of illness is frequent hand washing." Prevention doesn't get much easier than simply washing your hands. (www.webmd.com/cold-and-flu/cold-guide/cold-prevention-hand-washing)

Another step in the right direction regarding this issue is that it is becoming socially acceptable to ask others to wash their hands. For example, when doctors do not wash their hands when entering the exam room, they are now encouraging patients to remind them to do so.

There was a time when I was grocery shopping and approached the deli department. The employee was sweeping the floor and then emptied the dustpan into the garbage. He then came over and asked what he could get for me. I asked if he could please wash his hands before preparing my purchase. He kindly obliged, which is appropriate for public health. It's not always easy to ask others to wash their hands, but making the effort to do so can be vitally important to your health.

Teaching children proper hand washing should include three key components: explaining why hand washing is important to health, showing them how to wash hands correctly and teaching them how often and in which situations it should be a priority. Modeling appropriate hand washing to children will likely result in children repeating the behavior and being sick less often.

In addition to frequent hand washing, I also use a technique to reduce or eliminate the risk of becoming ill while in the presence of people who are sneezing or coughing. When someone nearby sneezes or coughs, I immediately turn and step away while exhaling. This reduces the risk of inhaling any airborne particles that may contaminate me. You can do this, too and teach your children to practice it.

Remember – Turn, Step, Exhale. You may have just avoided getting a cold or the flu – *or something even worse*!

CHAPTER 42

Being Healthy Can Keep You From Getting Hurt, On And Off The Job

"When safety is first, you last."

~ Author unknown

ACCORDING TO OSHA (the United States Department of Labor's Occupational Safety & Health Administration), "In addition to their social costs, workplace injuries and illnesses have a major impact on an employer's bottom line." (www.osha.gov)

OSHA explains that employers are currently paying almost $1 billion per week for direct workers' compensation costs. These costs are accrued in the form of both direct and indirect costs of workplace injuries and illnesses, which includes everything from workers' compensation payments, medical expenses, costs for legal services, training replacement employees, accident investigation and implementation of corrective measures, lost productivity, repairs of damaged equipment and property and costs associated with lower employee morale and absenteeism.

When I work with companies presenting wellness seminars, I obtain information regarding the status of their safety program, their wellness program, and most importantly, if they link them together. Sometimes companies have a strong safety program and make participation in the program mandatory. However, these same companies sometimes have no wellness program, or if they do have one, participation is voluntary. Emphasizing safety without also emphasizing wellness creates a disconnect between the two.

Safety and wellness should have a strong link, since they affect each other to a high extent. For example, an employee who works feeling tired, stressed and unwell (referred to as presenteeism) is much more likely to have an accident at work than an employee who is well rested, not stressed, alert and productive.

Focusing on our health reduces the risk of workplace injuries and saves companies a great deal of money. Employees remain healthy and fully employed. Another benefit is that employees who focus on health are not only happier, healthier and more productive, but they are also more likely to receive promotions and/or pay increases.

What areas of your health can you focus on to reduce the chance of suffering a work injury and help you be more productive?

CHAPTER 43

Reduce Chronic Stress

*"If you allow outside factors to stress you,
you will always be outnumbered."*

~ Carol Phillips

CHRONIC STRESS IS LIKE POISON in our bodies. Over time, festering stress robs us of our health.

Our bodies were designed to deal with a limited amount of stress; not nearly the amount most people deal with on a daily basis today. I use the following analogy when discussing stress with my clients. You purchase a beautiful white shirt for yourself. Over time, it becomes dull, and you wash it with a little bleach to make it look new again. A little occasional bleach in your laundry is comparable to a small, infrequent amount of stress, especially the healthy stress that comes with the excitement of, for example, interviewing for the job of your dreams.

However, if you wash the shirt every day in a large amount of bleach, the shirt will soon fall apart. Our bodies deteriorate when we allow too much stress to become part of our daily lives. Recognize the areas in your life that are stressful and find ways to change the stress you *can* control. Just as importantly, do not internalize the stress you *cannot* control.

Many of the ideas in this book are also great stress reducers. Here are a few more:

* In each situation, determine how much control you have over stress to help you come up with a plan to reduce it.

* Decide each day to find new ways, specific to what works for you, to deal with stress.

* Focus on being more organized if disorganization is an area that results in stress (for example, leave earlier for appointments to reduce stress caused by unexpected traffic).

* Use lists to reduce the amount of information you need to remember. Cross items off as you accomplish them. Determine what can wait until another day.

* Learn to say no when appropriate.

* Delegate duties to other people to reduce your work load.

* Analyze how you deal with problems and learn a new approach, if necessary.

* Accept that life isn't always fair; however, be fair to yourself and others.

Some changes can be simple but can have a profound effect on your health. For example, if the route you take to work is stressful due to traffic or other issues and a different route is less stressful and more scenic, it may be well worth the extra five minutes of drive time required to make that change.

Society is not going to slow down for us. We need to take control to eliminate chronic stress in our lives. As we reduce our stress, our health will improve.

What are the stressors in your life? Which ones are preventable with some action on your part?

Which ones are beyond your control but with some effort can be handled so you're not internalizing so much stress caused by these situations?

CHAPTER 44

Brainwork: The Way It's Designed To Function

"If you are depressed, you are living in the past.
If you are anxious, you are living in the future.
If you are at peace, you are living in the present."

~ *Lao Tzu*

WE LIVE IN A VERY BUSY SOCIETY where, with cell phones, computers and other electronic devices, it's easy to stay busy from the moment we get up until the moment we go to bed at night. Our brains were not designed to deal with this constant input of information.

Your brain operates much in the same way a computer does, taking in information, processing it and then providing an appropriate response. For example, we ask the computer for the address of a local restaurant (input), it tries to answer our question by taking that information and searching for an answer using the information previously stored in its memory, and then it spits out the answer. Our brain is built to work the same way (or rather, society designed a computer to mimic our brains.)

We are also designed to take in information, process it and provide information (solutions to problems, new ideas, taking part in a conversation and other actions). The challenge to our health happens when our brains are dealing with input all day long. Input overload is not healthy for our brains.

We need time to process information and provide feedback; otherwise, our brains are constantly overworked. If we don't take time to let our brains operate the way they're supposed to work, they will not perform efficiently and will become overwhelmed and unproductive.

Recognize times when you feel stressed because your life is overly busy, and you are dealing with multiple problems. The stressed feeling you're experiencing is your brain telling you to slow down so it can finish doing what it was designed to do. Prioritizing time to allow this to happen is one of the best things you can do for yourself.

Imagine if you kept putting one search after another into your computer without allowing it to process and give you the results you need. Your effort would be unproductive and your computer would eventually lock up. "Locking up" is what is happening to you when this area of your life is out of balance.

How can you incorporate more time into your day to let your brain process and provide you with the wonderful information you need?

CHAPTER 45

Positive Vs. Negative People In Your Life

"Don't feel guilty about purging people from your life who aren't healthy for you."

~ *Carol Phillips*

SPENDING TIME WITH PEOPLE who love and support us has a significant effect on our mental and physical health. Remember the saying about how we may not remember where we know someone from, or what they said to us, but we'll remember how they made us feel?

Our brain has a primal need to not only socialize with other people but also to associate with people who are kind and fair to us. We instinctively know it's healthy to work and play with people who will help us move in a positive direction in life. Otherwise, the conflicts and stress brought into our lives from people who don't have our best interests at heart stifle our growth.

When we have an awareness of being with positive, supportive people, we can relax and move in a productive direction. Positive, supportive people help in our efforts to make healthy decisions; negative, critical people tend to put roadblocks in our way. For example, if you want to quit smoking, a positive friend may help you find a distraction when you're tempted to have a cigarette. The positive friend will also cheer you on in your efforts.

On the other hand, a negative person will tempt you with a cigarette or smoke in your presence. They're also likely to make hurtful remarks when you have a setback.

Pay attention to everyone you associate with on a regular basis. In your mind, start putting them into either a mostly positive or mostly negative category. You may even discover that there are people who you thought were positive but, upon reflection, you realize, are not.

Remember, you shouldn't feel guilty about purging people from your life who aren't healthy for you. You may not easily distance yourself from family or friends who are toxic to your health, but usually it's necessary for your welfare.

Gravitate toward positive people who will have a positive effect on your life. The people you choose to spend the most time with *will* affect your health. Choose to spend your time with optimistic, supportive and encouraging people in order to maximize the effect on your health.

CHAPTER 46

Socialize

"Be yourself; everyone else is already taken."

~ Oscar Wilde

SOCIALIZING IS GOOD for the brain. Humans are social creatures. Personal interaction stimulates the brain and challenges our thought process. Simply exchanging a few words with a sales associate while you are running errands will spark enough activity in your brain to jump-start you into mental exercise mode. Yes, we need to exercise our brains as well as our bodies.

As different areas of health are often connected, socializing can benefit other areas of health besides brain function. For example, if you decided to join a hiking group to make new friends you would also be increasing your exercise. One healthy decision often automatically leads to another. Joining the hiking group to meet new friends gets the ball rolling, and the increase in physical activity that results from being part of the group helps the ball pick up speed.

A November 2008 *AARP Bulletin* article titled, "Friends Make You Smart," states: "Many recent studies document the positive effects of social interaction." The article explains that researchers are not certain what happens in the brain that results in the positive effects seen among the more socially engaged, but according to them, "it appears clear that close relationships and large social networks have a beneficial impact on memory and cognitive function as people age." (www.aarp.org/health/brain-health/info-11-2008/friends-are-good-for-your-brain.html)

These results are good news, especially in light of the high number of dementias in our country, including Alzheimer's disease. One of the early symptoms of Alzheimer's is refraining from socializing, which compounds the problems of the disease. Socializing is important at any age and seems to become crucial as we enter our senior years.

Have you ever watched the news when they interview people who have just turned 100 years old? Centenarians are typically asked what they feel is the secret to their longevity. I always listen for the pearls of wisdom that come from the mouths of these wonderful members of society. Frequently, one of their secrets is their continued efforts to socialize. Heeding their precious advice is certainly a healthy decision.

If someone asked you right now, "What are all the ways you socialize in a typical week or month?" What would be your answer? Is your current level of socialization sufficient to keep your brain stimulated to ensure health? Would the list be so long that the question of life balance comes into play?

Your personality type also plays a part in what is considered a healthy and balanced level of socializing. For example, the amount of socializing deemed healthy for an extroverted person may be far more than what an introverted person could handle. While one person may love being the social butterfly in large groups, another person may seek one-on-one socialization.

One way I challenge myself to be more social is to initiate conversation with strangers when I'm out running errands or when I'm in other situations in which I could easily choose to keep to myself. I purposely make eye contact, smile and say "Hi." Although being this outgoing is not always easy for me, I've met some very nice people this way, and I always feel better afterward. They seemed happier after our conversations, too.

Another simple way to socialize and meet new people at the same time is to invite a few friends out to do something fun and ask them to invite other people they know. A stranger is a friend you haven't met yet. Make it effortless to meet them.

What works for you? Do you have a healthy balance of socializing in your life? If you do, celebrate your efforts and share what works for you with others who may seem isolated. If you don't have a healthy balance, focus on what would interest you. People often find volunteering for a cause they support to be an easy first step. Lending a hand will give you many opportunities to socialize.

CHAPTER 47

Is There A Doctor In The House?

"The doctor of the future will give no medicine,
but will instruct his patient in the care of the human frame,
in diet and in the cause and prevention of disease."

~ *Thomas Edison*

REGULAR DOCTOR (or healthcare professional) visits give you an opportunity to discuss any health problems you may be having and learn important methods of treatment. Seeing your doctor regularly also gives you an opportunity to find out if you may be having a medical problem you're not aware of as well as learning new ways to maintain optimal health. Whether you choose a traditional doctor or alternative medicine, having an expert oversee your health and wellness and answer your questions is an important complement to your overall good health.

Although you don't have to memorize them, there are important numbers to know to prevent high blood pressure, heart disease, stroke, diabetes and other health problems. These numbers are obtained through regular biometric screenings and blood work. They include:

* Total cholesterol

* HDL ("good" cholesterol)

* LDL ("bad" cholesterol)

* Triglycerides

* Risk ratio

* Glucose

* Blood pressure

* Weight

* Waist circumference

Many health problems have no symptoms in the early stages, and some never have noticeable symptoms. Knowing your numbers and tracking them on a regular basis, helps you identify a problem before it becomes a serious health issue for you. Check with your healthcare professional to find out how often he or she recommends testing for you.

When you have blood work done, ask for the results in writing with the ranges included so you can easily keep track of your status in each area. Also, be sure to compare recent results to past results in order to monitor any changes in health. If you don't understand any part of your results, ask your healthcare professional to explain the results in easy-to-understand language so you can be your own best advocate.

CHAPTER 48

Put Yourself On Your Calendar First

"The key is not to prioritize what's on your schedule,
but to schedule your priorities."

~ Stephen Covey

WE ALL KNOW THE ANALOGY of putting your oxygen mask on first in an airplane emergency, which teaches you that you'll be much more capable of helping other people if you're taking care of yourself first. When you take time to prioritize your health, you'll have a much richer, healthier life.

If you have a history of putting yourself last, it's likely you "never get around" to taking care of yourself. Over time, ignoring your own wellness needs will almost certainly lead to major health problems. If you are not motivated to take care of you for your own sake, think about the feelings of other people who love you and want you to be healthy.

Claiming "me time" is like coming up for air after being underwater too long. Your brain will give you that "Ahhhh" feeling that tells you you're making a healthy decision. Making the wise choice to care for yourself has positive rewards, including reducing stress, reducing blood pressure, increasing concentration, reducing irritability, increasing your likelihood of making better decisions regarding many areas of your health and generally energizing your life with a sense of feeling more rested.

I'm challenging you to begin putting time for yourself on each day of your calendar before anything else is added to your agenda. Whether your "me time" takes the form of a 15-minute walk before work, going to bed 15 minutes earlier, taking 10 extra minutes at the grocery store to find healthier foods or 20 minutes of reading a book you enjoy, prioritizing time that contributes to your health sets up a pattern that becomes easier and easier to repeat. Claiming your "me time" also sets a great example for children.

Think of it this way: your calendar is YOUR calendar. Why put everyone and everything else on your calendar each day and not have any time for YOU scheduled? Put that oxygen mask on yourself first and you'll be much better able to breathe and handle the other demands of your day. Once you get used to making time for yourself on a regular basis, you'll look forward to those precious breaks in your schedule to spend time with YOU.

CHAPTER 49

Take Vacations (Or Staycations) On A Regular Basis

*"Today just get up and go
because yesterday you said tomorrow."*

~ Author unknown

WE ALL NEED A CHANGE OF SCENERY on a regular basis. Our brains and bodies become bored and tired of the same routine but also overwhelmed with the monotony. We become less and less productive when we don't listen to our instinct to take a break.

Have you noticed that when you return from a few days or weeks of being away, your brain seems to enjoy the experience of just being at home more than before your break? Your beautiful brain needs a change of surroundings and new things to see and do.

Changing the scenery doesn't have to involve spending a large amount of money. A retreat can be something as simple as driving an hour from home and hiking for a few hours or visiting friends you haven't seen in a while.

Vacations help remove you from the chronic stress in your life, especially the stressors you may not realize exist until you are physically and mentally removed for a time. A *Psychology*

Today article titled, "The Importance Of Vacations To Our Physical And Mental Health," confirms the significance of taking time away from our usual activities: "Chronic stress takes its toll in part on our body's ability to resist infection, maintain vital functions, and even ability to avoid injury." (www.psychologytoday.com)

Wait, before we go on, let's consider this list: 1. Resist infection, 2. Maintain vital functions, and 3. Avoid injury. How can you justify keeping your body at risk in these ways by living in a constant state of stress?

The article goes on to explain that simply being tired or stressed increases your likelihood of becoming ill, overworks your arteries, makes you more likely to have an accident, interferes with quality sleep, impairs digestion and may even alter the genetic material within your body's cells in a detrimental way.

As *Psychology Today* points out, "Mentally, not only do you become more irritable, depressed, and anxious, but your memory will become worse and you'll make poorer decisions. You'll also be less fun to be with, causing you to become more isolated, lonely and depressed."

Was there a time in your life when you didn't think you needed a break, but after taking one, you felt surprisingly refreshed, more positive and healthier? Responding in this way is a sign that your body was dealing with chronic stress and you weren't aware of the negative effects. The other extreme is when you know you're long overdue for a break. Listening to your body during these times is even more crucial because your health is already being significantly challenged.

When we take a break from our routines, we often spend more time with family and friends, which can positively affect our relationships. Just as we need to focus on our work to keep the occupational part of our lives healthy, we also need to have blocks of time to maintain healthy relationships. Most terminally ill people are quick to share their feelings of wishing they had spent more time with the people they love and not as much time working. Great advice!

Has it been too long since you gave your mind and body a true break from your usual routine? Taking time to recharge your batteries is not being lazy. The opposite is true: the effort will pay you in many health rewards. Now, look at your calendar and get excited about planning your next mind and body recharge!

CHAPTER 50

Is Your Work Fulfilling?

"You'll never feel perfectly ready,
but that doesn't mean you're not."

~ S.C. Lourie

DO YOU LOOK FORWARD TO going to work? Most people spend the majority of hours in their week doing the work of their chosen profession. If your work is an area of your life in which you find a sense of accomplishment and pride, your health will be affected in a positive way. However, if your work is unfulfilling, frustrating or stressful, your health will likely be negatively affected. To what degree the stress of your job impacts your health typically depends on the level of chronic stress caused by the situation.

Many different reasons can contribute to people feeling un-fulfilled and lethargic in their work environment. Some people may be doing work they don't feel passionate about; other people may work in fields they love, but the people with whom they work do not make the daily work experience a positive one. Or maybe, the company's culture is unhealthy.

Whatever the reason for work stress, the important question remains: overall, is this a healthy part of your life or an unhealthy part of your life? Do you feel truly valued at work?

Knowing the answer to this question is very important because it links directly to your health.

Maslow's Hierarchy of Needs, developed by psychologist Abraham Maslow in 1943, states that people are motivated by certain needs and these are achieved in a sequence from basic needs (air, food, drink, warmth, shelter, sex) to self-actualization needs (achieving self-fulfillment and peak experiences). The Hierarchy of Needs (usually diagramed using a pyramid) supports the belief that when we satisfy one level of needs, we are then motivated to move up and achieve the next higher level. Likewise, not achieving lower levels of needs keeps us from ascending to the next level.

One element of the hierarchy is job satisfaction. When we are in the lower stages of the pyramid, securing a job is enough to satisfy us. However, once we attain a higher level of growth, having any job is not enough, and we are motivated to hold a job where we feel fulfilled and purposeful in order to continue our growth toward self-actualization.

If you're not feeling satisfied in your work, what can you do to change the situation? Are there options available to you in your current position that you can use to improve the circumstances? For example, have you always wanted to go back to school but haven't explored what you need to do to make that goal a reality?

Oftentimes, taking the first step is all you need to do to create momentum that will lead to meaningful and rewarding change. *Suddenly, you'll be feeling better about life.* Forward movement in achieving your hierarchy is important to your health because it literally stimulates your brain to release *messages of hope and vitality* and motivates you to take action.

Where do you want *and need* to be and what will you do today to start your journey?

CHAPTER 51

Volunteer

*"Never underestimate your ability
to make someone else's life better
— even if you never know it."*

~ *Greg Louganis*

ENGAGING IN VOLUNTEER SERVICE has numerous physical and psychological benefits. When we aid others, we take a break from our own worries in order to focus on helping people, animals, the environment or causes in need.

When the causes we help matter deeply to us, then the gratification and the sense of fulfillment we gain grows to a higher level. Helping others simply for the joy of helping them rewards us with a sense of altruistic satisfaction. Volunteering not only makes us more satisfied mentally but brings with it numerous health benefits because often it is tied to a happier, healthier and more productive outlook on life.

When I suggest volunteering, a frequently asked question is, "Where can I volunteer?" Volunteering for a cause you feel strongly about is important. Your passion will not only give you a greater feeling of satisfaction from helping, but will also motivate you to continue to help and not become "too busy" to add a little service work to your schedule, which is easy to do in our busy society.

If you love animals and have a soft spot for those in need of good homes, you could volunteer at a local animal shelter. If you are passionate about wanting to find a cure for cancer, you could volunteer for the American Cancer Society. Ask family and friends if they know organizations in need of volunteers or you can look up volunteering in your area on the internet. You can even team up with a friend and use this as an opportunity to socialize and keep one another motivated to continue your volunteer efforts.

More often than not, when we are volunteering, our bodies are moving more than they would have been otherwise, which is hugely beneficial for our physical health. Volunteering can also reduce chronic stress and lower blood pressure.

Remember to keep life in balance. Volunteering is a great activity but only after you take care of yourself first. Giving too much will have a negative effect on your health. Taking care of yourself first will give you the health and energy you need to give more to others. Then everyone wins!

CHAPTER 52

Be Kind:
To Yourself And Others

"No act of kindness, however small, is ever wasted."

~ Aesop

I'VE SAVED THE BEST FOR LAST. I believe being a kind person, not only to others but also to yourself, contributes *significantly* to your overall health and wellness. Making an effort to be kind in every thought and gesture gives you a different perspective of the world. Immediately following an act of kindness, your mental and physical stress decreases. Time seems to slow down and positive thoughts and energies flow into your life.

When we practice kindness, we are forced to take stock of where we are in life regarding our own contentment. If it's difficult for us to be kind to others, the challenge we feel can be an indication that we have unresolved issues we need to face, which also contributes to our chronic stress. Being kind to others has numerous benefits to our own health, besides the benefits realized by the recipient. Being kind:

* Reduces blood pressure
* Enhances mood

* Distracts us from our problems

* Exercises the social part of our brains

* Helps release "feel good" hormones

* Reduces depression

* Increases longevity

Focus on finding positive attributes about other people instead of concentrating on what you perceive to be negative. Shifting your focus can improve your own health by inspiring within you a more positive outlook and reducing the stress that comes with having a negative view of others. Focusing on the positives also opens the door to your capability to be more compassionate in countless situations, which will then lead to healthier interactions and relationships.

Try this experiment: choose a day to look for the good in every person and every situation you encounter. Take each negative thought that comes into your mind and consciously dismiss it. Replace it with something positive. After a full day of changing your thinking, how did this process benefit you? How did it benefit others?

Keeping a positive frame of mind does not include letting people take advantage of you because that would not be healthy. However, in numerous situations, a positive mindset about others and yourself can have a huge impact on your overall health and happiness.

I find practicing random acts of kindness to be hugely beneficial to my overall health and wellness. Each day, I am on the lookout for situations in which I can help others. Most of the time, the opportunities take an incredibly small amount of my time but give me great satisfaction. For example, helping a mother who is struggling to open the door of a building while pushing a stroller; sending a quick supportive email to a colleague who is having a bad day; or allowing someone who seems in a hurry to move ahead of me in line. Helping others helps me to feel happy, healthy and productive.

Think of how you would treat someone if he or she was your best friend and you loved each other unconditionally. Think of how you would take care of them, protect them and defend them. Now, start treating yourself and others as your best friends and you'll have a much happier, healthier and more productive life.

Best of luck on your journey!
I know you will do amazing things with your life!

~ Carol Phillips

AFTERWORD

Introducing: The Gravity Technique™

Years ago, I had an incident at work in which I began to choke on a piece of hard candy. My immediate reaction was my brain telling me the best way to handle the situation. The message was clear: stay calm and use gravity and force to expel the object from my throat. I knew that if I could get more air into my lungs through my nose first, without further lodging the object, I would have a greater chance of expelling the object. In addition, I knew if I didn't get the object out on the first try, I could be in serious trouble.

I stayed calm. I bent at the waist to get my head and neck lower than my lungs. Before trying to expel the object, I slowly breathed in through my nose in an attempt to get more air into my lungs to increase the chance of expelling the object. I realized that the blockage must not be very far down because I was getting air into my lungs. Then, with all my might, I used my core muscles and blew as hard as possible out of my mouth to expel the air from my lungs, in the hope that the piece of candy would become dislodged. It worked and the piece of candy flew out of my mouth with more force than I anticipated, much like a cork being forced out of a collapsible bottle.

Years later, I began teaching CPR and First Aid classes and noticed the focus on the Heimlich maneuver, which has saved countless lives. However, this technique typically uses another person to perform the maneuver. The advice usually given for people who are alone and choking is to "throw yourself over the back of a chair" to try to mimic the Heimlich maneuver.

In my experience in health and wellness work, I have observed situations in which animals sometimes seem to make better choices than humans make. The common denominator in those instances was that animals tend to follow their immediate gut instinct, whereas humans can overthink situations or panic and not respond in a logical way. In an emergency, the difference between a logical and instinctive response and an emotional panicked response can mean the difference between life and death.

Picture a cat that is trying to get something out of its throat. The animal automatically puts its head down toward the floor and focuses totally on tensing its entire core and pushing the air out of its lungs to expel the object. The cat is responding instinctively. The instinct to use gravity to help one's efforts may be an effective technique for people to use when faced with a choking situation in which no one is present to help. Think of the experience I had and recall how effectively The Gravity Technique™ worked for me – it probably saved my life.

Using The Gravity Technique™ may be helpful if someone is alone and choking. The likelihood of expelling the object from a person's throat may increase if he got down on his hands and knees and positioned his throat lower than his lungs. This position allows gravity to help, instead of hinder, the situation.

An additional benefit of this technique is that if a choking victim becomes unconscious, he is already close to the floor, thereby reducing the chance of becoming injured, which often happens when a choking person is standing at the time he becomes unconscious. One of the biggest concerns of becoming unconsciousness while standing is a possible head injury that can subsequently occur from the fall.

I developed The Gravity Technique™ in honor of my brother, who tragically died at the age of eleven months from choking on a balloon.

I can take no responsibility for anyone who uses this technique. But I can share that in my situation, I followed my gut instinct and it worked. I share it in the hope that it may help others.

Other actions that may help before or during an emergency:

* When calling Emergency Services (or 911), make sure the address number is clearly visible on the outside of your house or building. If your house or building is not visible from the road, having the number on your mailbox at the end of the driveway can save critical time.

* If you're alone and are having an emergency, try to get to a landline phone and dial 911 so help is on the way. Sometimes using a landline, as opposed to your cell phone, can increase the ability of emergency crews to see your exact location immediately. Even if you can't speak, the dispatcher will likely see your location and send help. Your cell phone may also work if the GPS feature is on and accurate.

* If you are able to unlock or open an entrance door, your chance of getting help quickly increases. If you're alone and choking and are able, dialing 911 and then getting outside where people may be able to see and help you may also increase your chance of survival.

* Have all your personal information readily available for emergency and hospital personnel. I created a medical emergency form, which can be updated as needed. I keep a copy on my refrigerator in a "911" magnetic sleeve and a copy in my purse. You can also give copies to your emergency contacts.

My form contains the following information:

* Name

* Address

* Phone number

* Date of birth

* Medical conditions

* Allergies and drug sensitivities

* Special instructions (Wear glasses or contact lenses? Have pets at home that need someone assigned to take care of them?)

* Medication table (with meds listed down the left column; and dosage, frequency, reason and prescribing physician listed across horizontally)

* Emergency contacts (names, relationship, addresses and phone numbers)

* Physicians (names, addresses and phone numbers)

* Information regarding durable power of attorney, if applicable

* Date form was last updated

In an emergency, it is *much easier* to hand the form to emergency personnel than it is to try to remember all the information or try to retrieve it from several sources. This time is much better spent focusing on the emergency at hand. Depending on the emergency, you may not even have the opportunity to obtain the information if it's not immediately available.

A free, downloadable template of this form is available on my website at www.CoachCarolPhillips.com.

ABOUT CAROL PHILLIPS

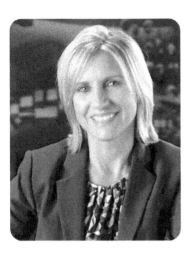

Carol Phillips is a national health and wellness expert with 25 years experience in the field. As an energetic health coach, author, speaker and consultant, she has helped thousands of people improve their health through her seminars and workshops. Her consulting work helps companies increase their return on investment through improvement of their employee wellness programs and increases their bottom line by educating and motivating employees to prioritize their health and wellness.

Carol is also a certified personal trainer, a CPR and First Aid instructor and a Smoke Cessation facilitator. She was one of New Hampshire's first Wellness Coordinators when Governor Lynch issued an Executive Order designed to promote health and wellness to NH State employees and their families. Carol holds degrees in Exercise Science and Health Education, graduating number one in her class and winning numerous awards.

A NOTE FROM CAROL

I'd love to hear your success stories and your tips for simple and easy ways to health. I welcome you to email me at:

carol@HealthDesignNH.com

Please put "SUCCESS" on the subject line. Due to the volume of correspondence, I may not be able to provide a personal response, so I thank you in advance.

———————

Book Carol for your next corporate event:
carol@HealthDesignNH.com

Bulk book order rates available by contacting the author at carol@HealthDesignNH.com.

CONNECT WITH CAROL PHILLIPS ONLINE:

www.CoachCarolPhillips.com

Facebook
www.facebook.com/carolphillipsauthor

Twitter
www.twitter.com/carolphillips52

LinkedIn
www.linkedin.com/pub/carol-phillips

Pinterest
www.pinterest.com/cphillips52

Book Carol for your next corporate event:
carol@HealthDesignNH.com

REFERENCES

Additional health information
is available at the following websites:

WebMD
www.WebMD.com

Mayo Clinic
www.MayoClinic.org

Centers for Disease Control and Prevention
www.cdc.gov

Healthfinder
www.HealthFinder.gov

U.S. Food and Drug Administration
www.fda.gov